FOR THE
LOVE
OF
GOD

**A CHRONICLE OF
FAITH THROUGH SUFFERING**

FOR THE
LOVE
OF
GOD

A CHRONICLE OF
FAITH THROUGH SUFFERING

John Wagner

FOR THE LOVE OF GOD
A CHRONICLE OF FAITH THROUGH SUFFERING

© 2023 by John Wagner

All rights reserved. No portion of this book may be reproduced, stored in a retrieval system, or transmitted in any form or by any means, electronic or mechanical, including photocopying, recording, or by an information storage and retrieval system - except by a reviewer who may quote brief passages in a review to be printed in a magazine or newspaper - without permission in writing from the author.

Cover design and interior layout by Uberwriters, LLC.
www.uberwriters.com

John Wagner's portrait photo by Kerry Quade, Moments to Memories Photography LLC
www.mtomphotography.com

All Scripture quotations, unless otherwise indicated, are taken from the Holy Bible, New American Standard Bible®, copyright © 1960, 1962, 1963, 1968, 1971, 1972, 1973, 1975, 1977, 1995, 2020 by The Lockman Foundation A Corporation Not for Profit La Habra, California. Used by permission. All Rights Reserved

Scripture quotations marked (NIV) are taken from the Holy Bible, New International Version®, NIV®. Copyright © 1973, 1978, 1984, 2011 by Biblica, Inc.™ Used by permission of Zondervan. All rights reserved worldwide. www.zondervan.com The "NIV" and "New International Version" are trademarks registered in the United States Patent and Trademark Office by Biblica, Inc.™

Scripture quotations marked (NLT) are taken from the Holy Bible, New Living Translation, copyright © 1996, 2004, 2015 by Tyndale House Foundation. Used by permission of Tyndale House Publishers, Inc., Carol Stream, Illinois 60188. All rights reserved.

Scripture quotations marked (MSG) are taken from THE MESSAGE, copyright © 1993, 2002, 2018 by Eugene H. Peterson. Used by permission of NavPress. All rights reserved. Represented by Tyndale House Publishers, Inc.

ISBN 978-1-7352174-0-6 paperback
ISBN 978-1-7352174-1-3 eBook

Dedication

For my wonderful wife, Mary
and
To all of God's children who struggle with faith.

Contents

Preface .... *ix*

Chapter 1: Sowing the Seeds 1
Chapter 2: ABCs and 123s 11
Chapter 3: A Turning Point 17
Chapter 4: Drifting 25
Chapter 5: Rollercoaster 33
Chapter 6: God's Timing 43
Chapter 7: For Better or for Worse 55
Chapter 8: And Baby Makes Three 63
Chapter 9: The Breaking Point 73
Chapter 10: Swimming Upstream 81
Chapter 11: Contagious Pessimism 89
Chapter 12: An Unexpected Gift 95
Chapter 13: Defeat in Victory 105
Chapter 14: Walking on Water 113
Chapter 15: Ambrotose 121
Chapter 16: Western Let Down 129
Chapter 17: Embedded and Undetectable 135
Chapter 18: The Disease That Never Was 143

Chapter 19: Into the Storm 151

Chapter 20: Desires of the Heart 161

Chapter 21: Dangers of the Heart 167

Chapter 22: God's Love Provides 177

Chapter 23: Strangers in a Strange Land 187

Chapter 24: A Change of Season 197

Chapter 25: Energy Healing 207

Chapter 26: Skeptical and Cautious 217

Chapter 27: Remedies 227

Author's Note *237*

Preface

Does confusion about God and His plan for your life ever get in the way of your love for Him? Unfortunately, I've experienced this for much of my life. Trials and disappointments have continually tried to pull me away from Him, but even with all that has gone wrong, my love for Him has only deepened. I truly love Him with all my heart, and despite life's many difficulties, I know He loves me immensely, too.

My deep love for God didn't come easily. I've had a life full of physical and emotional challenges exacerbated by deep feelings of failure. In my own head, I failed my mom by not persevering through difficulties in the ways she expected, my dad by not being the athlete he had once been, and my brother by being unable to counter his physical attacks against me. Most of all, I failed myself when I couldn't learn to read and write like my classmates. No matter how hard I tried, it seemed like I was constantly disappointing those around me, and mostly myself.

Along the way, I reasoned that if I was discouraging so many here on Earth, I certainly must be displeasing God, too. So, I spent a lot of time contemplating how to stop being such a failure. I usually came to the same conclusion: I just had to try harder—do more, do better. Then others would love me more. Then God would love me more, and when He loved me more, He would give me a better life.

Years passed, and despite considerable effort, my circumstances didn't improve. I reasoned that this was because I hadn't yet tried hard enough, done enough, or performed well enough. I still didn't feel respected by others and certainly didn't feel it for myself, either. Moreover, to make matters worse, physical challenges had begun to add to the emotional baggage I'd been dragging around for so long. Above it all, I was dogged by the feeling that I wasn't just inadequate to the people closest to me on Earth, but also to God because He still hadn't helped me out of my misery. In fact, it seemed like He was allowing me to fall even deeper into it.

My story is about how God changed my life—how He helped me find respect, love, and happiness. It's a story of how He saved me—not by taking my hardships away but by increasing their impact so much that there was nothing else to do but completely give myself to Him. It was both harder and easier than I ever thought it could be.

Chapter 1

Sowing the Seeds

Lord, how many are Your works! In wisdom You have made them all; The Earth is full of Your possessions.
Psalm 104:24

I'm a very typical guy. I'm middle-class and middle-aged. I don't have a fancy job or a fancy house. I have a wife, some kids, a dog, and a small home in a small town in the Midwest. I was born the youngest son of a farmer and his wife on a farm in Pickett, Wisconsin. By the time I came along, my oldest brothers and sister had already moved out on their own, so there were just Mom, Dad and five kids left on the farm. Dad was often gone selling crop insurance, so my older brother, Paul, and I were left in charge of the farm chores a lot of the time. It was a pretty big responsibility for relatively young, naïve boys.

I didn't appreciate it as I should have at the time, but when I reflect on my time on the farm, I'm in awe of its beauty, especially in the summertime. We had a big front yard with tall maple trees lining the road and a couple of acres of woods at the back of the house. Our homestead was perfect for a young kid to get lost for a couple of hours. After the morning chores were done, I often roamed through the woods or walked in the tall grasses around the fields, returning home only to grab some lunch before heading back out to adventure some more. I spent so much time outside that it wasn't uncommon for Mom to use a match head to remove ticks found in various places on my body that had already embedded themselves quite deeply into my skin.

My mom had a large flower garden on the west side of the house. Any time she had a spare moment, you would find her gardening—although when she was in there, she probably didn't want anyone to find her. That was her safe haven: a time to forget everything and get away. She loved her garden and was known for her ability to cultivate a beautiful assortment of blossoms. We loved it, too, albeit from afar.

On the east side of the house, Mom had a vegetable garden the same size as the flower garden. Since we lived on a farm and didn't need to grow corn, peas, or beans there, Mom focused instead on a large raspberry patch, a smaller patch of strawberries, and a few cucumbers and other vegetables.

While Mom took care of the house and the gardens on the north side of the road, the south side belonged to Dad. The barns, the machinery, and the fields located there were in his domain. Like Mom's flower gardens, Dad's fields had their own kind of beauty. The gently curving hills were arranged in tidy rows of corn, peas, wheat, and alfalfa whose colors changed with the seasons—from the light green burst of new growth to deeper hues of the mature crops to finally the golden, brown tones of drying plants before the fields eventually laid barren before us throughout the winter months.

One of the rituals on the farm every spring was picking stones. This was a process of preparing the field before any planting could happen. Every year, large stones would make their way to the top layer of the soil. Dad would hook up a flatbed wagon to the back of the tractor and gather the kids to walk beside it, chucking stones upon it as they were found. I still can't believe how many rocks arose from that dirt every spring!

Stone picking may not have been our favorite event, but it was always a profitable occasion for my mom. She loved it when we found large, flat stones that could be used to develop the walking path she was creating through her little piece of paradise. Each approved stone was lovingly placed just so, appearing somehow like it had been there forever. Because it meant so much to her, we were glad whenever we found a stone we thought she could use. It always felt great when we got a cheer of approval from Mom.

Life on the farm was fascinating in so many ways. One of my favorite memories was waking to the sound of the pea pickers and corn pickers approaching in the late night or early morning hours. I would hop out of bed and run to the window to watch the lights of the mighty machinery proceeding toward our fields. I couldn't help but feel in awe of the important events like this that took place right outside the four walls of our little home.

Dad's barn typically housed about twenty cows and three to five calves. The milk house was attached to the barn. All the milking equipment was kept here, along with the milk, which was stored in a large tank until the milk truck came to pick it up. Half of the upper part of the barn stored hay to feed the cattle, and straw for their bedding was held in the other half. Dad also had two other hay barns, a grain shed, and an equipment shed.

Loitering between the barn and field were usually a couple of cats. Most felines on the farm would come and go with little notice. Some were hit by cars, others were caught in the fan belt when the car was started on a cold winter's day (since they'd snuggled under the hood near the warm motor in an attempt to keep themselves warm), and some were likely chased out in the occasional turf fight. One cat stuck around more than the others and littered many kittens during her reign on our homestead. Pussy, as we creatively named her, was Queen of Mousing. Still, she was as loving a creature to the people in her domain as she was tyrannical to the rodents in her kingdom. Almost every time I saw her, she had a helpless rodent dangling from her mouth. Then half an hour later, she'd rub against my legs or curl up in my lap, purring contentedly. I don't know if it was her prowess or her affection that made such a big impact on me. It was likely both.

Along with the cats, we had dogs on the farm, too. The first one I remember was Silky. Silky was a great cow dog. When it was time to bring in the cattle, she would run around them, chasing them toward the barn and nagging them until they were where they were supposed to be. One afternoon, I walked into the barn and noticed Silky lying on the ground near an empty stanchion. She had foam coming out of her mouth. I started over to her, but she began to growl at me, letting me know I shouldn't come any nearer. I didn't understand what was wrong with her at the time, but I recognized that she wanted me to stay away. I ran up to the house and got my dad. When Dad saw her, he told me to get out and stay out. I watched from afar as he strode right to the house and came back with his gun. A few seconds later, I heard a lone shot. After that, I never saw Silky again. Looking back, I reasoned that Silky had growled at me because she knew she was dangerous, that her growl was a message of love. She kept me away so I would stay safe. I've always regretted that I couldn't have repaid her kindness by helping her, too.

In addition to our farm animals and pets, there were plenty of other critters on and around the farm. We shared the land with salamanders, badgers, foxes, and white-tailed deer. Bald eagles occasionally flew overhead, and for part of one summer, a family of skunks lived under the front porch. There were always mice, too—lots of them! In case you're wondering, mouse holes like those seen in cartoons really do exist, and they don't look nearly as quaint as what you see on TV! We had mouse holes in the baseboards of our home and also in drawers, cupboards, and floors. Conversations in our house were often accentuated by scurrying mice feet and the occasional SNAP of a mousetrap. None of us thought much of it—it's just how it was.

A telling aspect of our family dynamic and hierarchy was evident at the dinner table. Our kitchen floor had a pretty severe slant, and our large dining table stood in the middle. If anyone knocked a drink over, it would run down the table and into the lap of the person sitting at the lowest end. I was the youngest in the household, so that was my seat. I learned to stay alert and to move pretty quickly!

For all the beauty around me as a child, some parts were not so pleasant. I didn't realize the dysfunction then as much as I do now because I was just a kid and didn't know any better. The darkness it cast upon my early years, though, had a definite impact on my life.

Mom and Dad had been married for about twenty-three years before I came along. The way Mom always told it, she never loved my father and, in fact, had preferred another. Since the other man was a Protestant and she was Catholic, they were basically forbidden to be together. Not so lucky for her, Dad was

Catholic. Nevertheless, both sets of parents had no concerns with the union, so they were engaged and soon married. In later years, we learned that Mom really had loved Dad at first and had chosen him over the other. Either her current reality had erased her memory of the event, or she simply kept the truth from us to emphasize her displeasure. Either way, she lived most of her married life in regret.

On the other hand, my father loved my mom from the moment he first met her, and he continued to love her until he died. His affection, though, was darkened by a personality flaw that caused him to act in very controlling ways. I don't think he meant to be that way but was trying to project himself as confident and wise while deep down feeling quite the opposite. Anger had been building between my mom and dad long before I was born. By the time I was old enough to recognize it, my dad was making unreasonable demands upon my mom. She, in turn, was critical and short-tempered back at him. They fought continually and were miserable. Although most of their disagreements blend together into one bleak picture in my mind, I do recall one in particular that reflects how the rest of the family learned to live with the constant upheaval caused by their arguments. The kids were all in the kitchen as Mom was preparing supper. We were practically salivating as the aroma of a freshly baked pizza began to waft through the space, and all of us waited with probably not-so-quiet anticipation of gobbling down a few pieces. Then Dad came into the room and must have said or done something that really set Mom off. Suddenly, Mom slid her hand under the hot pie, aimed, and threw it right in his face. We all watched and probably gasped a little as we saw it hit the mark perfectly, then drop facedown on the floor. I still remember feeling a pang of deep regret that, of all the things she could have thrown, she'd chosen one of my favorite foods at a time when I was so hungry. I don't recall what actually happened next. I suspect that Mom and Dad went their separate ways until they cooled down. As for my brother and sisters and I, we probably did our best to salvage at least a bit of that meal, even if it exceeded the five-second "safe-to-eat-off-the-floor" rule. After all, we were used to turbulence in our home and had learned to make do even amid such chaos.

Despite the considerable conflict between Mom and Dad, they had one thing in common: they had grown up through some pretty rough times and, as a result, were pretty tough-minded themselves. As newlyweds, they started out with absolutely nothing: no electricity, no running water, and no gas heat. They'd come a long way by the time I arrived, but their toughness remained.

During my childhood, we lived on a decent farm and had a house with electricity, gas heat, and running water. Even with those things, though, Mom and Dad always looked for ways to save money. One thing they did was heat just the main floor of the house. Because the house wasn't insulated, those of us with bedrooms upstairs (my brother, my three sisters, and I) got to experience plenty of freezing nights. When it was bedtime, we always got under the covers quickly and didn't dare move in fear of touching a part of a bed sheet we hadn't touched before because it would have been cold! In the morning, it was common to see our breath in the frigid air of the bedroom. Waking up with a cold nose, however, was just the beginning: once morning had arrived, my brother and I knew we were expected downstairs and then out in the barn to get started on our chores. There was no other way to do it but quickly. At least we'd have a bit of reprieve downstairs, where it was warmer, before we headed outside into the crisp air and across the road to the barn.

It wasn't much better in the summer, but for the opposite reason. Now it was so hot upstairs all we could do was sweat it out. I remember we all had to share one fan—the girls sleeping in one room around the corner from my brother and me would all fight for ownership of it. Mom often settled the controversy by putting the fan in one window to blow the warm air outside. Her goal was to create a vacuum through the house, pulling the cooler nighttime air in through one window and pushing the warm air out the other. I spent more than a few hours by my window trying to grasp this philosophy, but I have to admit I never did buy into it because I could never feel it.

Although Mom was tough, we knew she loved us. She told us so and frequently gave us hugs. Still, most of the time, she didn't mind displaying her heavy hand, either. Once, after begging her for quite some time, she agreed to go outside to play catch with me. She'd never done this before, so I was very excited. We set ourselves up in front of the flower garden, and she started to throw to me. We were only out there for a couple of minutes before she threw a grounder that bounced up and hit me in the nose. Blood started to run down my face. I fell to my knees and started to cry. I wanted Mom to come and take care of me, but when I looked up, I saw her walking back to the house. I staggered after her, crying now because I didn't understand why she was leaving. She ignored me for a bit, then turned around and sharply said to me, "You finish the play! You pick up the ball and finish the play!" Then she left.

Another memorable example of my mom's tough attitude occurred when I was about ten. My brother and his friends were up in the silo, and I was trying to tag along, as usual. Paul was throwing silage down to feed the cows for the night, and he knew I was climbing up behind him. He waited until I got about halfway up the ladder and started throwing the silage on top of me. In an attempt to stop being such an easy target, I hurried up to where he and his friends were. As I popped up near where he was standing, he was swinging his pitchfork to send down another batch of silage. Unfortunately, the tines of the huge fork pierced right into my knee, knocked me off my feet, and caused me to fall about ten feet onto the silage at the bottom of the silo. Ironically, the fall was the least of my problems: the real issue was the agony I felt because of the gaping, bloody hole below my knee.

I struggled up and out of the silo through its opening into the barn and hobbled to the house to show Mom. I couldn't find her at first, but after a few minutes, I saw her approaching the road in the car. She turned into the driveway to park but wasn't even out of the car yet when I stumbled over to her, lifted my leg to show her my wound, and told her what my brother had done. Her reaction was not what I expected (but then again, maybe it was). Instead of reaching out to comfort and care for me, assuring me that all would be okay and that my brother would get the punishment he deserved, she looked me squarely in the eye and asked, without any sympathy or concern, if I'd finished my chores. When, through my tears, I shook my head and mumbled that I hadn't, she coldly directed me to ". . . put a Band-Aid on it and get back to the barn!" So that's what I did. I bandaged it as well as I could on my own and headed back to work. I don't recall her ever saying anything to my brother about it, and she never even mentioned it to me again. When I talked to my brother many years later, he was still amazed that he'd gotten away without any consequence for his actions. So was I.

In fairness, Mom's firmness resulted from a life in which she had to be tough to survive. She had to grit her teeth and get through many difficult things, as did many others who lived during that period. In addition, she felt stuck in a world of discontent stemming from her unhappiness with my dad and the physical and emotional dysregulation that often occurs during the later middle-aged years of a woman's life. Still, her response hurt me deeply for many, many years. I needed a champion in my corner that day. When she couldn't be that for me, the pain in my heart was more intense than the pain below my knee.

Dad was a pretty tough guy, too. He once needed someone to paint the stanchions for the cows. I was only about nine at the time, and like most kids that age, painting sounded like a lot of fun. I begged and begged him for the job. Finally, Dad had had enough of my pestering and agreed to let me do it. Of course, I was ready to be done after about ten minutes. When I broke the news to Dad, he made it clear that this wasn't how it would go. He'd given me the job, and I was expected to do it until it was done—and done right. I don't remember how long it actually took to accomplish the task, but it felt like it took me all summer. I never begged for another job after that.

I tell these stories because of their impact on my life. God had blessed me by placing me in such a beautiful world, yet allowed me to experience a great deal of distress at the same time. Ironically, much of my life reflected this juxtaposition. As a result, I developed a highly disciplined personality that enabled me to persevere through intense physical or emotional challenges and stick with challenges longer than most to achieve results. Unfortunately, my never-let-up, don't-feel-just-do perspective ultimately contributed to unrealistic personal expectations that affected my emotional well-being.

Looking back on my life, I can now see how God shaped it to prepare me for the life He had planned for me. I'm lucky that as far back as I can remember, I knew the basics about Him: He was in Heaven, He was powerful, and He loved me. Still one day, as I wandered around the yard doing typical little-kid things, a particularly deep thought popped into my head. Who made God?

I wondered. And if somebody made Him, who made that guy? There was only one thing to do—ask Mom. "He was just always here," she told me. Well, that wasn't very satisfying. I asked the same thing or some version of it again and again until she finally brought the conversation to a close by reassuring me that, one day, I would know the answer. So, for now, I would have to accept that it is just that way.

I recall pondering this mysterious concept for days, maybe even weeks. Looking back at it now, I think this was God's way of introducing Himself to me. I guess everyone has a moment or two like this. Some choose to ignore it or, for whatever reason, don't pursue it. Others, like me, become overwhelmed by its complexity. Like most, I couldn't understand His plan for my life while it was happening, but for some reason, I recognized that I'd need discipline to get through what was and what was to come.

My feelings about and toward God would change over the years, and despite the rosy beginnings, my feelings weren't always positive. I often felt abandoned, which was often disappointing and sometimes made me outright angry. Eventually, my continual difficulties caused me to consider that God must be punishing me for something. I searched my mind to recall what I might have done to make Him mad at me. When unable to land upon anything of consequence, I began to wonder if I was being made to suffer the consequence of something someone else had done. Maybe my mom, dad, brother, sister, or someone else was unable to pay a price for Him, so I was expected to do so for them. There seemed to be no other explanation. God was being extremely hard on me for some reason or another. If only I could figure out why and fix it so my problems would go away. Ironically, even in my darkest days, I never felt that there wasn't a God or that God wasn't present in my life—I always knew He was there; I just didn't know what He was doing.

Chapter 2

ABCs and 123s

For I consider that the sufferings of this present time are not worthy to be compared with the glory that is to be revealed to us. For the eagerly awaiting creation waits for the revealing of the sons and daughters of God. For the creation was subjected to futility, not willingly, but because of Him who subjected it, in hope that the creation itself also will be set free from its slavery to corruption into the freedom of the glory of the children of God.
Romans 8:18-21

When I was about four or five years old, I became severely ill. Mom and Dad finally took me to see a doctor after waiting a while for my health to return to normal on its own, as tough farmers did in those days. By that time, I was weak and dehydrated, and I couldn't keep anything down—not even the smallest sip of water. The doctor who saw me was concerned enough to admit me to the hospital immediately. I don't remember much about it except for waking up at one point and, to my surprise, noticing I had plastic tubes going in and out of different parts of my body.

For some reason, even today, no one seems to know what the diagnosis was or what exactly had been done to help me. Other than receiving multiple doses of antibiotics, the details are sketchy. Years later, Dad would admit on a few different occasions there was considerable concern that I wouldn't make it. Although the doctors sent me home and everyone considered that I was healed, I've always wondered if these events marked a turning point in my life—a turn from what would have been a "normal," healthy one to something very different.

Within the year, I was back in the hospital. This time, I was admitted so I could have my tonsils removed. The thought was that the constant sore throats, earaches, and other related issues I was experiencing could be resolved by getting rid of those troublesome tonsils. So out they came. After arriving home from the hospital, I experienced some unusual and extensive bleeding, so I was taken back. After a day or so, the medical staff was satisfied they'd been able to stop the bleeding because, once again, they sent me home.

The following year, I was ready to start kindergarten. I was excited and a little nervous. Though if I could have foreseen the future, I should have been a lot more hesitant because this place called school would drastically change my life. Kindergarten started well. I had no trouble with milk break, nap time, coloring, sharing, and playing with my classmates. I recall once overhearing my teacher tell my mom that I was one of the brightest kids in the class. Maybe the teacher was just saying that because I was standing right beside her, or perhaps it was something she told all the parents to make them and their children feel good about themselves. Regardless, those words meant a lot to me, and I carried them close to my heart for quite some time.

When I think back to those days, I realize how much I wanted to feel validated, to be recognized in a special way. It was already important for me to feel smart and successful. As a kindergartener, I thought I could do anything with my life. Maybe I could even be a doctor one day. Or a scientist. Even though I was still very young, I began making big plans for my future. I could hardly wait: I was going to really BE somebody!

By the time first grade rolled around, my teacher's compliment from kindergarten was still in my mind. I had no reason to doubt that I'd succeed at school again, yet first grade turned out to be very different from kindergarten. First, although we still had a milk break, there was no nap time. Second, while we still colored, shared, and played with friends, we did much less of it than we'd done the previous year. Instead, we were expected to sit still and listen to the teacher much of the time. We were also told to do tasks that required multiple steps without reminders or repeated directions. Third, there was reading: I just couldn't make the connections everyone else seemed able to make with letters, sounds, and words.

This new school version was so different from the one I'd championed the year before. It took a lot of work in first grade to pay attention as closely and for as long as needed to understand the lesson or the directions. I tried to tell myself to "Just focus!" (or a six-year-old's version of that) repeatedly, but my mind wandered off only seconds later to yesterday's baseball game or that afternoon's adventures in the woods. In addition, I wasn't able to remember things that other kids seemed able to recall without any trouble. Whether it was single ideas or a series of events, no matter how hard I tried, I couldn't bring the ideas back into my mind.

In addition to mental challenges, I also began to have physical ones. I'd get frequent bloody noses—really severe ones. I think I could have filled half a glass with the amount of blood I'd lose each time. Also, my ears began to ring, and the ringing would continue for hours. A third physical symptom was an extreme reaction to ragweed. I recall one time walking through the back forty property on the farm when I must have come in contact with some ragweed. Before I even left the field, my eyes were swollen shut. I could only cry out for help because I couldn't find my way back home. Thankfully Dad heard me and was able to take me there. Soon after, I developed a similar reaction to hay. I quickly developed welts at its point of contact, even if I just brushed slightly against it. In addition, I would often have severe sneezing fits due to the hay or ragweed pollen in the air which could go on for ten minutes at a time, especially in the fall.

Next, I began to experience periods where I would lose my vision for a few seconds. Sometimes stars and lines appeared right before everything else became black, but at other times, the rest of my vision remained while the stars and lines appeared along with it. I know that people sometimes have this experience when they get up abruptly, but in my case, it would happen even if I was just sitting.

Mental and physical challenges weren't my only problem during this time in my life. I also began having trouble with my brother. Paul was four years older than me, and for whatever reason, he wasn't a very loving brother—even though I really could have used one. I looked up to him, though, because I needed someone to look up to and because he demanded it. When I was in first grade, Paul was in fifth. He was probably dealing with a lot of issues at school and with his friends during that time, leading to at least some degree of stress that he tried to relieve by bullying me. He also had an overwhelming amount of responsibility on the farm, which had to have been incredibly difficult for him. Dad was gone most afternoons selling crop insurance, so Paul, at age twelve, was in charge of the bulk of the farm chores. Knowing how hard Mom was on me, she was likely just as hard on Paul, so he was probably struggling with that too. All of this didn't make his treatment of me acceptable, but when I think back to those days, it helped me justify his attitude and actions.

My biggest challenge with Paul was that he was domineering. He began to ask, bribe, or demand I do things that time and time again would be to my detriment. For example, one afternoon while we waited for the bus to pick us up from school, Paul and his classmate pitted the classmate's brother and me against each other in a boxing match. I was positioned in one corner of the foyer in the front of school while the other boy stood across from me in the other corner. On a signal from our brothers, we were told to punch each other relentlessly until the bus came. Ironically, I remember feeling pretty good despite the punches I was getting when I heard Paul shouting words of encouragement and praise above the frenzy. Later on, I recognized this as manipulation: he would compliment and high-five me as if he was proud of me, which ultimately led me to do the next dumb thing he wanted. On the other hand, I quickly learned that doing what he wanted was safer than refusing to do it. If I didn't do what he demanded, he would attack me in some way as a consequence.

It likely isn't surprising that my mental and physical issues, along with my brother's bullying, made it nearly impossible for me to be successful in the classroom. In addition, most of the schoolwork made absolutely no sense to me, so it wasn't long before I was academically far behind my first-grade peers. Thankfully, my class was part of a first and second-grade split class, and my sister, Sara, was actually in the classroom with me. She watched over me and helped me whenever she could, but unfortunately, it wasn't enough. By May, it was obvious that I hadn't mastered the first-grade material. That meant only one thing: I would have to repeat first grade.

The second time through first grade was even worse for me. Academic challenges were no easier than they'd been the first time around. In addition, my mental and physical ailments were just as bad, if not worse. Moreover, because I was constantly failing, I was an emotional wreck. My former classmates—now second graders—teased me about being left behind. I didn't even have my sister in my classroom anymore, so I was really lost.

I cried many days before school and many nights in anticipation of the next. Probably due to sheer self-preservation, I could at least keep from crying while I was at school. Even though I tried not to show it, others must have known how inadequate I felt because I was picked on regularly. Part of the reason I'd been chosen as a target likely had something to do with my brother, Paul, who'd offended many at the school because of his rough attitude. Although he'd left for middle school that year, some remembered him, made the connection between the two of us, and were ready to get revenge on the Wagner that remained.

It felt to me like there was no end to the torment. It was mostly the same few who antagonized me again and again. They called me names, pushed me, and even held me down after school until my bus left. Ironically, it wasn't the idea of missing the bus that worried me, but instead, what Mom would say when she got the call that she'd have to come and get me. I even remember wanting to walk home so she wouldn't have to be bothered, but since it was about eight miles to my house, I was afraid I would get lost, which would likely disappoint her even more.

To avoid missing the bus due to the bullying, causing Mom to have to come and get me, I made a plan. I hid in the school or somewhere safe around the building until the bus came into sight, and then I ran as fast as possible to get on before anyone could bother me. This ploy must have been pretty successful because it's the way I remember waiting for the bus most days.

I don't know why it never occurred to me to stand up to, fight back, or tell an adult about the abuse. Instead, I just tried to stay one step ahead of my persecutors, which was mentally and physically exhausting, especially on top of everything else going on in my life at that time. When May came back around the end of my second year in first grade, I was hardly farther ahead than the year before, and since you can't flunk a kid twice in the same grade, I was promoted. Ironically, the idea of flunking kids must have gone out of favor at some point after my repeat of first grade because even though I didn't do any better after that point, they passed me on to the next one almost automatically each time. Maybe they wanted to get me out of school as much as I wanted to get out.

Chapter 3

A Turning Point

Have I not commanded you? Be strong and courageous! Do not be terrified nor dismayed, for the Lord your God is with you wherever you go.
Joshua 1:9

I was eleven and in fifth grade when my mom and dad divorced. Back then, in our small, Midwestern town, not many people got divorced, so I didn't really know what divorce was. It didn't even enter my head that my mom might leave my dad even though they rarely got along. One day, Mom just called the younger kids together and said, "I'm leaving Dad, and you guys are going with me." When Mom decided to do something, she just did it. This news stirred mixed emotions in me. On the one hand, I was extremely happy to be leaving the farm because my allergies had become so intense. In addition, my chore list had steadily increased as I'd aged, so that I now had a pretty big load. Furthermore, even though I spent a lot of time with my dad in the barn and the fields, I didn't have a very deep connection with him, so leaving him wasn't a big deal for me. I didn't even feel bad for him—I just felt nothing. On the other hand, I felt really sad for Paul because Mom wasn't planning to bring him along. She didn't love him any less—it was just a business decision of sorts. She knew Dad would never be able to do everything on the farm on his own, so leaving Paul with him would give him the help he'd need so he wouldn't lose the farm.

I knew Paul was going to have a hard time with this new situation. Now he'd have even more work than before, which was already a lot. Even more difficult would be the challenge of living alone with Dad. They both had very strong personalities: Paul didn't like to be bossed around, and Dad always wanted control. I'd already witnessed many arguments between them. I could only imagine what it would be like when it was just the two of them together all the time.

That same day, Mom, Jane, Sara, and I moved to Grandpa's house not far away, where we stayed for three months. After that, Mom rented an apartment for us in Ripon, which was only about a fifteen-minute drive from the farm. My sisters were excited about moving to town, which was closer to their friends and provided more opportunities for them to do the kind of things that girls their age liked to do. I also found a lot in town that made life pretty interesting, but without Paul there with us, I couldn't help but feel like a part of me was missing. Although we weren't very far apart, we didn't see each other very often. After all, we were in different schools, and Mom wasn't interested in going anywhere near Dad. Paul had always been so physically and verbally aggressive toward me, but I felt a bond with him nonetheless. I think he felt as bad about our separation as I did, but it was even worse for him because the fracture wasn't just between him and me; it was between him and his mom, too. He was a tough guy, so he never showed it or said anything about it, but being left behind on the farm must have been incredibly confusing and painful for Paul.

As time passed and Mom's anger toward Dad lightened, she occasionally took us back to the farm to help Dad with rock-picking or some other big task. Sometimes we just went there to visit Paul. I know I didn't miss his bullying, but I did miss him. I know, too, he missed me because we both cried the first time we saw each other after our first separation. Sure, Paul had been my worst enemy, but he was my brother. It was hard to come to terms with the idea that our relationship would never be the same.

At about this time, Billy Joel released a song called Only the Good Die Young.[1] The song wasn't complimentary to Christians,

---

[1] Joel, Billy. 1978. *Only the Good Die Young.* Vinyl. Written by Billy Joel. New York: Columbia Records. https://en.wikipedia.org/wiki/Only_the_Good_Die_Young.

but I didn't understand enough about it then to recognize why. I just really liked its catchy beat, so I often sang along to some of the words when it came on the radio. After I'd heard it a few times, I was drawn to one line in particular: "Aw, (your mother) never cared for me, but did she ever say a prayer for me?" It made me think of how I should have said prayers for others instead of criticizing them. I probably didn't know the word "hypocrite" at that time, but I realized that I was behaving like one when I did this.

My behavior at that time wasn't pleasing to God, and it wasn't even pleasing to me, yet I still struggle with some of the same things today. Thankfully, God continues to remind me what He expects from me through Bible verses, examples from others, or even pangs of realization that seem to come out of nowhere. I first recognized then what I still know today: that my first reaction to almost everything should be to pray. When I am irritated by others, when people are unkind to me, when I am overwhelmed, when I feel incapable, when I don't know how I am going to make it, I need to pray. Prayer can make things better for others and better for me, too. It can change things—even if it's only my perspective.

When sixth grade came around, it was time to leave the small Catholic school I had attended since kindergarten to join a large group of strangers my age in the public school system. For some reason, most of my Catholic school friends were not in my classes in this new public school, so I felt very alone. To further my insecurity, I had been assigned to some special-ed classes, where other kids like me, who struggled with learning, had also been placed. Clearly, this wasn't a badge of honor, and everybody knew it. It was very embarrassing to be there, so I hid out in the bathroom until the bell rang and then snuck into the special-ed classroom when the hallways had emptied so no one would see me enter the class. I guess I was trying to salvage a little of my pride. It's hard to have status with your classmates when you're not smart enough to be in the same room with them.

At least while I was in the special-ed classroom, I wasn't being teased. That wasn't the case when I was in the regular classroom. Whereas before, when only the older children had picked on me, now kids my own age were doing so too. I'm not sure if they did this because they knew I was in special classes or if my shy, quiet demeanor made me an easy target. Maybe they were just cruel. Likely it occurred—or at least continued to occur—because I simply didn't fight back or tell anyone about it.

While my peers' words were hurtful, it was the teachers' reprimands concerning what they thought was my lack of effort that were the most caustic. Nothing was farther from the truth. I *was* trying. No one put more pressure on me than the pressure I put on myself. I wanted to be bright and respected by my classmates, my teachers, my mother and father, my siblings, and most of all, God. When you only get Fs, however, it doesn't seem very likely. The thing is, I was quickly approaching my limit for this kind of treatment.

Despite all my difficulties in school that year, I found a niche for myself where I could excel: in the boxing ring. Boxing taught me a lot. First, I learned I could take a punch. Second, I learned I could give a punch. Third, I felt no fear about either one. To me, we were both in the ring for one reason: to hit the other guy. If you were to talk with me before or after a match, you would undeniably meet a different person than the one who was in the ring. Don't get me wrong—I was always concerned about my opponent when I was done, and I truly wanted the best for him. Boxing was merely an opportunity for me to overcome my reality as the kid who always got picked on, the one whose academic challenges never seemed to cease. It wasn't personal between the other kid in the ring and me—he was just an obstacle standing in the way of my achievement.

I won most of my fights, but it would be one of my losses that taught me the most. The match was held in my hometown, and although I wasn't told anything about my opponent beforehand, I later learned the guy I was scheduled to box was a year older than I was. He also had a reputation for being pretty good. That was my initial response when I stepped into the ring and looked across at him for the first time. I could tell that he was the better fighter. He was bigger and stronger, appeared to be two or three years older, and looked like he could beat the daylights out of me. I found out later that our coaches had arranged the match because neither of us had an opponent in our own weight class that day. It didn't seem like a very sensible or sensitive decision from my coach, but maybe he knew more about me than I did at that time.

I remember how differently the two of us behaved before the match: one was jumping up and down, throwing punches in the air and bouncing from side to side as if foreseeing an easy victory; the other one stood flat-footed, with his arms drooping by his sides, looking at his coach as if the man was nuts and wondering just how he might be able to get out of this fight.

I know I said that I was never scared when boxing, but I'm going to amend that statement to say I was scared *just once*. Actually, I was more than scared—I was *terrified!* Suddenly, the bell rang, and I braced myself as I awaited my opponent's charge, which would surely annihilate me. My challenger didn't come, however. So, tentatively, I moved toward him and met him in the middle of the ring.

For a moment, I thought the fight might not go as badly as I'd initially thought. Unfortunately, it did. I became this guy's punching bag that day. Right from the start, he began to throw hard, accurate punches. He was fast, he was big, and he was in control. I was not, not, and not, respectively. One thing I did well, though, was absorb the punches. Blow after blow, I somehow stayed on my feet. Throughout round one, I never went down, and for me, that was a victory! I don't remember what my coach told me when I returned to my corner, and I can't even tell you how I felt other than to say I was completely exhausted. Who knew that getting hit that many times would be so tiring?

Before I was ready, it was time for round two. It went pretty much the same way as the first, and I really began to hurt; it felt like some ribs were broken, and probably my nose too. Finally, after what seemed like a lifetime, I heard the bell that marked the end of round two. I still hadn't gone down, but I was in bad shape!

When I returned to my corner, I collapsed onto my chair. I had nothing left to give (or so I thought), and I didn't care if everyone in the place could see that. One person at least noticed, however—my coach. I'm not sure if he grabbed me to focus my attention or if he just yelled in my face, but he had a message for me: "You have all day to sleep tomorrow, but for right now, you go out there and give it everything you've got to win the third round!"

That line has stayed with me all my life. It seems simple, but his message was big and bold. It was just like when my mom snapped at me after I started crying when I was hit in the face with the baseball: "You have to finish the play!" She had shown me no sympathy then, and my coach wasn't showing me any now. So even if I had broken ribs, a broken nose, or any other problem, I needed to move past my feelings. After all, I had all day to sleep tomorrow, but right then, I had to go out there and give it everything I had to win the third round!

When the bell rang to mark the beginning of the round, I jumped off my chair, beat my opponent to the middle of the ring, and went after him with everything I had. By this time, he was also getting a little tired. I felt the adrenaline pumping through me, and although I didn't know if I could keep it up the whole round, I knew that I had what it took for the moment. I laid into him and didn't stop. I can still recall the look on my opponent's face as if he was thinking, *What the heck just happened here? I was in total control of this fight, but now this guy seems possessed!* When the third round was over, it was obvious I'd won the round, and that was good enough for me. For a moment, I felt like Rocky Balboa.

I didn't win the match, but I had proven to myself I wasn't a nothing. In fact, even in defeat, I felt like a champion! There are certain events in your life that define you, and this was one for me.

By eighth grade, I'd finally reached my limit for abuse. One day on the football field during recess, I was being picked on again. That day (as on most days), the bully was the group's ringleader. He was doing his usual routine: calling me names, pushing me, and so on. He had no idea what was coming, and I guess I didn't either. I suddenly reached my breaking point.

When he got close, without warning, I snapped and punched him square in the face with every ounce of my weight. I then grabbed him, pulled him to the ground, and continued punching him as hard as I could. We rolled around and tussled for quite a bit until, at some point, we returned to our feet, broke apart, and just stared a long, cold stare between us. He turned and walked away first. I could see my blows had been very effective, leaving him with two swollen eyes and numerous bruises. I had gotten him pretty good.

A Turning Point

After the fight, we both went back into school, but something had changed. Throughout the rest of the day, people I had never spoken with before and people I didn't even know came over to me to give me high fives, pat me on the back, or say something positive to me. I was suddenly being treated the opposite of how I'd expected to be treated. Even those who'd been pals with the bully congratulated me. Before I knew it, I was part of The Crowd. Naturally, it felt a lot better to be part of the crowd than out of it, but at the same time, I felt that God probably wasn't as happy about my new status as I portrayed myself to be.

In high school, I still had allergies, nosebleeds, earaches, and sore throats, but overall, things weren't as bad as they'd been in elementary and middle school. I guess that's because kids in high school are more focused on themselves than others. Of course, my success against the bully that year had given me a status that caused others to leave me alone. Still, it's hard to go into a place every day knowing that you are going to fail, which was the situation I faced. It didn't help that back in those days, teachers often posted test scores on the classroom door after an exam or big assignment. I always knew where to look to find my name: at the bottom of the list. At the end of the day, everyone knew three things about those scores: where their name was, who was at the top, and who was at the bottom. My academic failures were never a secret.

Despite some victories along the way that helped lighten the load, I continued to be an emotional wreck throughout high school. I cried privately more than I ever wanted to let on, and as you might imagine, I had little to no self-confidence. My hope for the future was extremely dim. Even so, despite my grim circumstances, I couldn't take my eyes off a girl in the same grade and had high hopes that one day we'd get together. She had a natural prettiness that drew me to her, and she was also down-to-earth and very kind. I was afraid to approach her for a long time simply because rejection from her would have shattered me.

Most Saturday afternoons or nights, the kids in our class would meet on a back road at the edge of town to hang out. It was during one of these parties that—to my shock—the girl I'd admired for so long approached me and asked me to take a walk. Of course, I agreed, and before I knew it, she was holding my hand. Her hand in mine was the best feeling I'd experienced up to that point in my life.

I don't think I let go of her hand all day. Nevertheless, after I got home that night, I was overcome with insecurity. All I could think about was how long it would take her to find out who I really was. How long would it be before she realized she was too good for me: too smart, too good-looking, and too far out of my league? Surely, if she somehow didn't realize this herself, someone else would tell her. In my mind, being dumped by her was inevitable. Still, I craved every second I could spend with her.

We stayed together for several days and then for several weeks. After a couple of months, I slowly started to believe that maybe she really did like me, that she saw something in me that others couldn't. Then, in the third month of our relationship, when we were together at a party on the Saturday before Christmas, she told me that our relationship was over. We had been there for less than ten minutes.

My eyes immediately filled with tears, and before I knew it, I found myself bawling in front of everyone. I cried long and hard, and *everyone* saw it. When I got home, I continued to cry for days. During my relationship with this girl, I felt important for the first time in my life. Why had God given me this joy if His plan was just to take it away from me? Was He really that cruel? Or was it my fault? Did I do something wrong to displease Him? Had I been too happy? Too proud? Too carefree? I didn't have any answers, so I resolved to do what I had always done in situations like this: try harder to please Him.

I never had another girlfriend during my time in high school, but I did have a lot of good friends. From the outside, I probably looked like I was doing fine, but on the inside, that was far from the truth. I spent a lot of time alone, often listening to melancholy music or mentally composing my own sad songs.

The worst part was when my friends began to plan for college, and a life of bigger and better things, while I had no options beyond my own hometown. Luckily, I had no idea that what I had in store was even worse than I could have imagined.

Chapter 4

Drifting

*Trust in the Lord with all your heart and
do not lean on your own understanding.
In all your ways acknowledge Him, and
He will make your paths straight.*
Proverbs 3:5-6

Life didn't get any easier after high school. For a short time, I worked at the Pickett Co-op gas station, selling cigarettes and gum while I watched the gas pumps. I was also required to sign some farmers' names on the back of their checks because many of them couldn't read or write. It's ironic that I, of all people, was given the task of writing for them. It should have been an easy job, but because I couldn't spell myself and had a terrible memory, I didn't know how to spell their names, even if I could recall them. This really irritated the farmers. I think my inability to write their names, the same names they couldn't even write themselves—was doubly hurtful to them. After enough of them complained to management, I was let go.

For the next several years, I floundered around doing odd jobs and working at the local canning factory during harvest season. Nothing permanent stuck, though, as I was either let go like at the co-op, or the seasonal work ended like at the canning factory. During that time, I either lived in Ripon with my mom or on the farm with my dad. My dad was no longer livestock farming at that time, so I didn't have to do any chores, which kept me from being affected by the hay and other grain allergies that had made living there so difficult for me when I was younger. I went back and forth between the houses without any real sense of purpose. My parents both knew something had to change and began to kick me out little by little—more with their words than anything else. It didn't matter that I was paying them rent; they were tough-minded people, and I hadn't established myself as they felt I should have by that point in my life. Eventually, they made it so uncomfortable for me that I would rather have slept on the curb than in one of their homes. It wasn't that they didn't care about me; rather, it was because they did. It was clearly time to be on my own.

I was lucky, I guess, that my Uncle Gene owned a small construction company. One evening, while at a bar, I began talking to my brother's friend, who had been working with my uncle. While we sat together, I told him about my situation, and he suggested I join him on a job in Racine, a city nearly 100 miles away. He said I could start working on the site the next day. Since I didn't have any other options at that point, I decided to give it a try. My brother's friend then drove me home, where I threw a few things into a bag, and we headed to Racine. At sunrise the next day, I became a construction worker.

Uncle Gene ran a non-union shop, so we frequently worked twelve or more hours a day for two weeks at a stretch before having a day off. It's safe to say that anyone who could get a better job wouldn't be working for Uncle Gene because the pay was far too low for the danger involved, as well as the demanding work and long hours. My impression of them on that first day was that they were pretty rough and tough, and when night came, their demeanor was even more unsettling.

Since the construction company would be on site for an extended period of time in this location, Uncle Gene had purchased a dilapidated house near the job site for the workers to share. It was evident from the moment I set foot on the premises that none of its inhabitants were interested in creating a cozy living experience there. There was no furniture, no TV, and no pictures on the wall. Blankets used as beds were strewn on the floor all over the house, and it was always dark and cold inside.

For some reason, there were always lots of people coming in and out of the house once the workday had ended. Some of the people were guys I worked with, but there were many I'd never even seen before. It wasn't unusual for me to come home to find miscellaneous friends, girlfriends, or wives sitting around on the blankets. Once I came home to find someone I didn't even know being intimate with his lady friend on the blankets where I slept. It made me physically ill to think about it later that night as I lay there trying to fall asleep, but my only recourse was to push it out of my mind.

You'd think the guys would take it easy after their shift ended, but as hard they worked during the day, they played even harder at night. Most times, they'd go to a local bar to eat and drink right after work. Sometimes they'd go to one and stay there all night. On other nights they'd move from one to another until one or two o'clock at night, then stumble home, fall onto their blanket and sleep for a few hours until the call came at five or six o'clock to get back to work. I wanted to fit in, so I tried to join them once a week, but I had a really hard time keeping up. Anytime I drank, even if I only had a fraction of the beers they did, I had a terrible hangover the next day, which took several days to clear up. In addition, it was incredibly difficult for me to survive on such a small amount of sleep.

One day, when one of my co-workers saw how hard I struggled to have the energy I needed for the job, he offered me some pills that he described as uppers. He said they would just keep me awake and wouldn't hurt me, so I tried them. Well, he was right that they did help my energy, but they also made my face feel numb, and my hair feel like it was standing straight up. It was a horribly uncomfortable feeling. At the time, I couldn't understand why it was so difficult for me to mentally, emotionally, and physically match what the others were doing.

Working for a construction company at any time can be dangerous and tiring, and in the mid-eighties, health and safety were not enforced like it is today. We never wore a safety harness when we worked up high, including when we walked along the steel beams forming the skeleton at the roof of a structure. Although I definitely had a fear of falling, I was committed to doing whatever my job needed, so I took chances and pressured myself to walk the steel beams with the best of them. The risks I took weren't smart, but they made me look fearless and earn the respect of others. Once again, God's hand protected me during so many dangerous moments.

After the job in Racine was complete, our construction company worked on many other sites around the state. They all involved long hours of grueling work in dangerous situations. On one occasion, we were in Green Bay building a warehouse. Over time, it dawned on me that I hadn't seen my partner for a while. I asked around to see if anyone knew where he had gone, but no one had any information. After the word got out that he was missing, an awful realization dawned on us. One crew member carefully scooted near the edge of the roof where my partner had last been seen and looked down. There was his body on the concrete slab far below, his body intact but his head surrounded by a small pool of blood. We all knew that there wasn't much chance of him having survived the fall, and our fears were soon confirmed.

That night as I replayed the events of the day in my mind, I was confused by how nonchalant I felt about my partner's death. I was typically a very emotional person, so I didn't understand why I wasn't responding as I usually might to such an awful situation. Even when I first saw him lying on the pavement, I had very little feeling—either good or bad. Why hadn't I been more unhappy, fearful, or mad? Suddenly it became clear to me: I wasn't sad for him—I was envious of him. I wished I had been the one to leave this life because I simply didn't want to struggle through it anymore. Life was just too overwhelming and too depressing.

The next day, most of the workers seemed to get back to work as if nothing had happened, but I was still considering things pretty deeply. Now that I'd clarified for myself that I'd have preferred to be the one to have fallen to my death, I began to wonder whether, if I had, God would have deemed me worthy enough to join Him in Heaven. I didn't doubt my love for Him nor His love for me, but I wasn't sure that the way I'd lived my life would have enabled me to experience the fullness of His prize. Suddenly, I began to consider the danger of this job in a new light. It wasn't dying itself that bothered me, but the eternal consequence that I'd inherit if my end occurred before I'd proven to Him that I was worthy of it. This realization made one thing very clear: it was time to make some important changes in my life and, to improve my chances, it was time to get a new job.

Although I was highly motivated to find a new job, the process required a lot of courage. Whenever I went to a place of business to get an application, I always asked to take the form home rather than complete it on-site. I did this so I could look up the correct spelling of words and get help from someone if need be. At times, if I didn't know how to write something correctly, I just left that part of the application blank. I hated being reminded time and time again that I could barely read or write.

In the back of my mind, I was already beginning to worry that if I got a new job, I wouldn't be able to do what was required. I put a lot of pressure on myself not to look dumb or incompetent, which, given my circumstances, took a lot of effort. I hadn't worried about being successful when I'd begun working in the construction field because I was pretty strong and athletic and knew I could do physical labor, but how was I ever going to handle anything else? I tried to ignore the voice in my head, voicing the usual doubts: *Would I be able to meet expectations? Would there be reading, writing, or math that I couldn't do? What else might be thrown at me that I wouldn't be able to handle?*

After a few weeks of applying for different positions, I was hired at a local box manufacturing plant. As my first day of work neared, I began to regret leaving my previous job and contemplated just forgetting this new opportunity and going back there instead. I tried to reassure myself that the lifestyle I'd experienced during my time as a construction worker hadn't been so bad. I'd liked a lot of the guys, and I'd been pretty good at what I did, which didn't happen very often. Thankfully, though, my inner voice of reason was louder than my inner voice of fear. I put thoughts of returning to the construction business out of my mind and began to focus on this new opportunity.

My new bosses started me out slowly, so I was never overwhelmed. I caught on to what I needed to do without much difficulty, and management seemed to appreciate my work ethic. My self-confidence didn't skyrocket, but it didn't sink, either. I worked hard, never missed a day, and always tried to present myself in a positive light so that even if I didn't do well, management might want to keep me around anyway. My attitude, resilience, and work ethic did a lot for my self-esteem, which in turn seemed to make me feel a little better physically.

Things weren't perfect, however. There was some writing involved in this job, and it wasn't long before I made spelling mistakes, which my co-workers found quite humorous. In addition, I was always extremely tired, even though I often got twelve to thirteen hours of sleep a night. My emotions also continued to overwhelm me, just like when I was a kid.

After a year at the box manufacturing plant, I'd gained enough confidence to apply for jobs in my hometown that offered a little more money and improved benefits. Somehow my application was complete and accurate enough for me to land an interview at Creative Forming, a small plastics thermoforming plant. I was offered a job as a second-shift mechanic. I was scared out of my mind!

I was frightened because I knew nothing about thermoforming and didn't know the first thing about running big equipment. Worst of all, because I'd attended high school with several people who were employed there, I was embarrassed even before I started because of my reputation as a poor student. Failing once again in front of former classmates terrified me. I was worried sick that I'd made a big mistake!

The plant manager at Creative Forming normally did the hiring, but he'd been away during my interviews and wasn't the person who'd offered me the job. When he returned to find that someone had gone over his head by hiring me, he was not pleased. It didn't take long for me to feel his hostility—especially when things didn't go right. One such situation involved an arrangement I'd made when I was hired. The man who had given me the job had agreed to let me take a day off on the Friday of my first week to attend my niece's wedding. I had missed my grandpa's funeral (a man I'd greatly respected and loved) a few years earlier because of the commitment I'd felt to my job, which had bothered me for a long time afterward. I didn't want to make a mistake like that again. When the plant manager found out about the arrangement, he wasn't shy about showing his displeasure. I knew by his actions and words that he didn't believe there really was a wedding to attend, and he tried over and over again to get me to come clean. I somehow managed to shrug off the pressure and went to the wedding, all the while knowing that I was digging a hole for myself by doing so.

When I returned to work, the plant manager was even more hostile than before. He continually criticized me and tried to make my life difficult. It was as if he was doing everything possible to get me to quit. I saw it as a competition: Would he bully me so much that I would quit, or would I stay and continue to put up with his harassment? After six months, I was still there and was beginning to feel as if I had won. He had a trick up his sleeve, though, as he informed me one day that he was demoting me to the position of inspector/packer. Maybe he thought this would be the final straw for me. He didn't know me, though. I'd been dealing with difficulties all my life. I was persistent above just about everything else. I may have been humiliated and demoralized, but I was persistent. I don't know if he realized it yet or not, but I was going to win this battle.

In my new role, I focused on packing parts as quickly and efficiently as I could. I always arrived on time and didn't miss a single day. Once a week, I went to the plant manager's office to ask him how I was doing or to ask him how I could do better. I made it very clear by my efforts that I wanted my job as a mechanic back. It was a long road, but slowly it seemed like my nemesis was warming up to me. He'd consistently treated me miserably, but I continued to do my best to be an excellent employee. I slowly began to sense that his attitude toward me was softening.

Three months later, I was granted my job back as a mechanic. By that time, I think the plant manager actually liked me. Don't get me wrong. He was still tough on me, but I took every one of his suggestions to heart. Soon I discovered that because I was so intent on proving myself, I was putting more pressure on myself than he was putting on me.

I'd grown a lot during my time at Creative Forming, but there was still room for more growth. I continued to struggle with self-confidence, which caused me to overreact to comments or actions from those around me. When I should have just ignored or laughed at sarcastic words from my co-workers, I often snapped back with a few choice words of my own. At the time, I felt I needed to do this to defend myself, but it was a vicious cycle that continued to rear its ugly head for many years.

I was starting to feel more competent as a mechanic, however. I began to notice that there were times when I could problem-solve technical problems better than others. I guess I had a knack for envisioning how things worked together—or how they should work together—more easily than most. This was an incredible surprise, and perhaps the first time I felt a unique sense of worth.

Since my life seemed to be moving in a positive direction lately, I reckoned that God must be a little less dissatisfied with me than He'd been in the past. I began to hold out some hope He'd bring success to other parts of my life, too. I started thinking a lot about finding the right woman. I had been on a few dates but hadn't yet met anyone special. I was hopeful that God was pleased enough with me to help me with this task, too.

Chapter 5

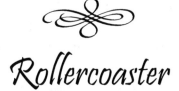

Rollercoaster

And the Lord is the one who is going ahead of you; He will be with you. He will not desert you or abandon you. Do not fear and do not be dismayed.
Deuteronomy 31:8

Getting my feet on the ground at work was such a great feeling, and my social life soon became more satisfying, too. One of the highlights of my summer was a recently-started tradition of traveling to the nearby state of Minnesota with some good friends to watch a three-game series between the Brewers and Twins. It was something I looked forward to every year.

I didn't know it then, but this year, the trip would be a little different than the others. On Saturday, after the second game of the series, we all headed to downtown Minneapolis to have some fun. We found a few bars and hung out there for several hours, talking and watching the crowd. Eventually, it got to be pretty late, but instead of heading straight back to the hotel, we decided to make one more stop at a little dive bar along the way. We found a table near the back to have our final few beers and wind down. A few minutes into the conversation, a girl came over and asked if I would dance with her. Some guy kept hitting on her, she said, and she thought she could get rid of him by acting like she was there with me. I didn't really care at that point—dancing with a pretty girl was just fine with me.

To continue the charade, we sat down together after we danced and acted like we were talking about the good times. Just talking with her was a good time for me. She was pretty, about the same age as me, and seemed to have a good personality. It didn't take much thought to realize that I'd landed in a pretty sweet situation. When I learned she was also a visitor to Minneapolis from the city of Appleton, Wisconsin, I couldn't believe my luck. Appleton was only a forty-five-minute drive from Ripon. We were practically neighbors! At Bar Time, she gave me her phone number, and I told her the name of our hotel with the hope that she and her friends would stop over to visit the following day.

My mystery girl never did stop by, and although I don't remember the specifics about the next day's game, I recall that the Brewers weren't too impressive, either. As my friends and I headed home, I felt very content. I'd had fun with my friends, connected with a pretty girl, and overall experienced a great escape from the daily grind. After a few days at home, though, I just couldn't shake the memories of the mystery girl. I still had her phone number—I just needed to find my courage. Eventually, I did. She seemed a little surprised to hear from me, and I was equally surprised when she agreed to go out with me!

We made plans to meet in Appleton and then travel to a nearby state park that was popular for its beauty and walking trails. I already knew that I liked her more than I should after such a short period of time. The day ended too quickly, and after we'd gone our separate ways, I couldn't stop thinking about her. I called her the next day and then the next, and pretty soon, it was just expected that we would be talking at some point every day. Each weekend, we made plans to get together, and every once in a while, we made plans for time together during the week, too.

She was the first person I'd really liked since high school. I'd gone on other dates since then but only occasionally, and there hadn't been anyone with whom I'd connected as well as I connected with her. At that point in my life, I wasn't just looking for an exciting short-term experience—I wanted a substantive long-term relationship. I wanted to find someone with common sense who was selfless and down-to-earth, but those characteristics seemed hard to find. The girl I'd dated in high school had those qualities, and this new girlfriend did, too. The fact that both were so good-looking was just a bonus!

The first couple months of this new relationship were nearly perfect. We had fun together, and I had never been so happy. In the back of my mind, though, I quickly began to fear that things were going a little too well and had a foreboding that this happiness would be short-lived. I soon began to doubt my worth and her perception of me: *Was I making enough money for her? Was my future bright enough to keep her interested?* It wasn't a mystery that I wasn't wealthy and that I was just a plant worker with a high school education. You don't have to be overly materialistic to want more than that in a life partner, so I wouldn't have been surprised—or even have blamed her—if she felt that way, too.

During this time, I also started to become especially conscious about how clearly and sensibly I was able to express my thoughts. I'd always known that my mind ran fast—so fast that words would often run on top of each other and fall out of my mouth in a jumble. Sometimes I'd still be speaking one thought while my mind was already on the next. It had been like that for me for as long as I could remember, so I'd learned how to compensate for it. Now, however, it seemed like my mind was racing even more quickly than before. As a result, it took greater concentration to organize my thoughts into words and then put them together into a logical sequence to express my thoughts. I hoped this wasn't as obvious to my new girlfriend as it was to me.

The problem was that the more I thought about it, the worse my thought and speech problems became.

By the third month of our relationship, things were still going well between us. We continued to enjoy each other's company, and there were no warning signs on the horizon. We'd had a minor disagreement here or there but never really fought. I was quick to write her a letter or card to tell her I loved her or to apologize for something whenever there was an occasion to do so. This was a dangerous move for me, given my tendency toward misspellings, so I was really careful to check things over thoroughly before sending her anything in writing. Nevertheless, it was bound to show up eventually—and one day, it did. In retrospect, I'd likely misspelled or had written things incorrectly before, but on this day, she finally brought it up.

For the Love of God

    I wanted to share my feelings for her and had decided to write her a poem. Even though writing it was risky, it was something that would have meant a lot to me, so I wanted to do it for her. I was very careful. First, I wrote out everything I had been feeling, and then I carefully examined the spelling of all the words. After I'd double and triple-checked them all, I wrote out the final copy. Before I sent the card, I hastily jotted a final thought, telling her I loved her with all my "hart." Then I put the card in the envelope and dropped it in the mail. I could hardly wait to see and hear her reaction.

    On our next date, I was anticipating an enthusiastic reaction to the poem I'd written. Unfortunately, her response was not what I'd hoped. One of the first things she did was ask me if I knew how to spell. I wasn't a liar, so I admitted the truth about how I'd struggled with reading and spelling and how I had been a miserably poor student in school. While I talked, she didn't say much, and she seemed very quiet the rest of the day, too. It was as if she was contemplating this newfound information about me. I, on the other hand, almost immediately began to try to make up for my shortcomings by going out of my way to say and do just the right thing for every moment and occasion. As much as I didn't want to think about what she was thinking, I couldn't help doing so and imagining the worst. *Was she disappointed? Embarrassed? Sad? Was she planning to say or do something big because of it? Would she really dump me because I didn't know how to spell "heart?"* By the end of the day, I was a nervous mess. It had been a long and gut-wrenching day for me, and she didn't give me any reason to feel any better before we parted ways that night.

    The following week was exhausting. Between anxious thoughts and numerous prayers for God to make everything okay between us, the weekend finally arrived, which would ultimately reveal if my true self was or was not acceptable to her. I expected the worst when I saw her, but was pleasantly surprised by her attitude. We got along very well that day and had a great time together. It was as if the previous dreadful weekend—or at least my perceptions of it—was just a bad dream. At one point, while sitting in a booth waiting for our food to arrive, she slid a napkin across the table upon which she had printed, "I love you!" My heart almost burst. Suddenly all couldn't have been more right in the world. She said she loved me! Me—with all my imperfections and struggles. Me—it was right there in black and white. It was by far the best date we'd had.

That date was also our last. Throughout the first part of the next week, all my attempts to contact her were in vain. At first, I thought she was just very busy. After all, she'd told me that she loved me. By Wednesday, however, when she hadn't answered the phone or returned any of my messages, I began to feel sick again with worry. On Friday, though, I was overjoyed when the phone rang, and it was her on the other end. Unfortunately, the conversation lasted only long enough for her to tell me that it was over. She didn't want to be with me any longer. She was done.

I was dumbfounded. *How had things changed so quickly? What had I done? What hadn't I done? If the issue was related to my misspelling in the poem the week before, why had the following weekend been so wonderful? How was it that she had just professed her love for me, but now she was dumping me?* To this day, I still don't know the answer to those questions. I tried many times to contact her to learn more but to no avail. Just like that, she was gone, and I was shattered.

I have always wondered if her telling me she loved me was her way of saying goodbye. Maybe she really did love me but had been pressured by others to do better: to find someone smarter, or richer, or more handsome. I don't know, and I likely never will on this earth. I want to think of her as loving me but having to move on because of outside influences that were too strong to ignore. Even if she was the one talking herself out of our relationship, I understood. Heck, if I were her, I would have probably done the same thing. We all want to marry up—or at least laterally, don't we? Being with me wouldn't have been either of those things.

After about a week, when it was clear things were broken off for good, depression like I had never experienced before settled over me like a dark, heavy blanket. I couldn't eat. I couldn't sleep. I couldn't move on. When she was with me, I'd felt like somebody important, and I'd become dependent on that. People seemed to look at me differently, and I had confidence like never before. Now she was gone, my self-worth had plummeted.

In my misery, I thought back to the other broken relationship that had meant so much to me in high school, as there were some important similarities. They had both lasted for about three months, had ended abruptly without any say on my behalf, and had wrecked my heart.

Then things got worse.

I became fixated, not only on the girl but on what it was about me that caused her disapproval. I should have tried harder. I should have done things differently. So I made a plan: I would get her back. I really believed that I could do it if I tried hard enough. I would impress her by proving my love for her. I would love her so much that there was nothing she could do but love me back. I did everything I could imagine. I sent her flowers, letters, and cards. I called her constantly to let her know I was thinking of her. I was thrilled when she would talk to me, albeit briefly, each time. Still, for some reason, she absolutely refused to see me. Over time, it became clear that my plan wasn't working. I was still desperate to have her back, but began to see what I was doing more closely resembled the actions of a stalker and less like what someone involved in a real-life relationship would do, and decided to let her go. When I did, though, I silently promised that I was doing this because I loved her, not because I'd stopped loving her and then stopped communicating with her altogether.

It's incredibly difficult to climb out of depression. Everything is bleak, and life appears hopeless. Consequently, in an attempt to find some relief, many turn to drinking, drugs, overeating, or sleeping. People with depression have little energy for anything other than to fold up in a dark corner with whatever short-term relief they can find. Sadly, many who are too tired or overwhelmed by the fight commit suicide. It's easy for people on the outside to mistake the actions of someone who is depressed as being selfish, but those with depression aren't doing it for attention or pity. They are just trying to make sense of their world and doing their best to deal with the continuous pain.

That's what I did, anyway. For two long years after the breakup, I tried to cope by sitting in the corner of my bedroom in an attempt to make sense of my life. It was dark in that corner, and it was also gloomy and uncomfortable—just like me. Although the pain was so severe that I'd considered suicide, it wasn't an option for me because I grew up believing I would go to hell if I did. I didn't know if that was true or not, but I sure didn't want to err and be on the wrong side of eternity.

Thankfully I never turned to drinking or drugs in my misery. I'd smoked marijuana a few times in the past, and my last experience with it was the reason I'd stayed away from it for good. I'd been with a friend one day when he took some out and invited me to smoke it with him. I smoked more of it that day than I ever had before. Suddenly, my heart began to feel like it was beating out of my chest, the walls looked like they were closing in on me, and the sound of someone's laughter rang eerily through my mind. I was so spooked by the experience that I recall lying down on the bed and pleading with God for help. I told Him that if He allowed me to make it through this situation alive and well, I would never smoke marijuana—or whatever it was—again. Having given my word to Him, I would never go back on it. So now, regardless of the hopelessness and despair I felt, smoking marijuana to help me cope wasn't something I was willing to consider.

I tried not to let on to my friends how depressed I was or even show it while I was at work. Although I lost twenty pounds during that time and wasn't the jolliest guy to be around, I put a lot of pressure on myself to act like I had my life together when I was in public. When I was home, however, I went right back to my corner to cry and ruminate through the same two questions: First, what had I done wrong? Second, when were things finally going to turn around for me?

Eventually, I stopped asking questions and instead began to plead with God. "Please bring her back to me," I begged. "Why would You let her go away?" Unfortunately, even though I begged Him constantly, He never seemed to hear me. I felt like Paul Newman in the movie Cool Hand Luke when, near the end of the film, Luke, the main character, enters the church and asks, "Is anyone in here?" Then, he begins to talk aloud as if to God:

> I know I got no call to ask for much, but even so, You got to admit You ain't dealt me no cards in a long time. From here, it looks like you got things fixed so I can never win out. Inside, outside . . . You made me like I am. So just where am I supposed to fit in? Old Man, I got to tell You, I started out pretty strong and fast, but it's beginning to get to me. When did it end? What do You got in mind for me? What do I do now? All right. All right. On my knees, asking

For the Love of God

... Yeah, that's what I thought. I guess I'm pretty tough to deal with, huh? A hard case, yeah. I guess I got to find my own way[2].

Luke's words might as well have been my own because I, too, felt like things hadn't been fair in my life. I just kept playing a losing hand. At the end of that scene in the movie, Luke got down on his knees and looked up to Heaven. He probably didn't expect a response from God but certainly hoped for one. The audience is left with the impression that God was silent—that Luke was on his own. That's exactly how I felt, too. I felt abandoned. I wondered why God wasn't helping me. Not once did it occur to me that He was actually doing what was best for me. I never considered that He was preparing the way for someone in my life who was just right for me.

***

For two years, my depression and the routine I'd established to try to deal with it was the same: I came home from work, sat down in the corner of my room, and peppered God with questions. "Why am I so dumb?" "Why do I have to struggle so much?" "Why did You take her from me?" I basically spent the time criticizing Him. I neither saw nor gave Him credit for anything that went well in my life. I just complained and spoke to Him with anger and despair.

Then, one sunny summer day, when I was on my knees, praying for God to fix my life or take me out of it, there was suddenly an incredible, thunderous clap that shook the room. A loud voice commanded me to "GET UP!" I looked around bewildered, as if trying to see who had come through my apartment door and into my bedroom, but just as suddenly as the words had come, the room was still. I was all alone, but I felt very much that I was in the presence of My Father. I knew immediately what He wanted of me: to stop acting as if life was such a miserable curse; to stop moaning and whining about how bad things were in my life; and where I didn't feel blessed, to take action to help myself instead of sitting on my knees and begging for Him to do everything for me.

The experience literally gave me goosebumps, but even more importantly, it gave me the push I needed to break free and go forward. After that day, I never sat or knelt in that corner again.

---

2   Rosenberg, Stuart, dir. 1967. Cool Hand Luke. United States: Warner Bros.

It was time to move on. Before, I'd thought God wanted me on my knees, praying to Him to bring me relief. From that point on, though, I knew He wanted something different from me. He wanted me to do more than just beg Him for help. He wanted me to do my part, too. It was almost as if He was telling me, "Put a Band-Aid on it and get back to the barn!" as my mom had said so many years before. His command to "GET UP!!" wasn't offensive to me at all—it was comforting. I had finally heard from Him. He'd confirmed to me that He was there, that He was listening, and that He was talking to *me!* I felt embraced, knew what I had to do, and was happy to get started.

Slowly I became more active outside of my apartment. I played golf, hung out with my friends, and even went on a few dates. At work, I continued to grow as a mechanical problem-solver and was able to make adjustments to improve production that others didn't recognize. Engineers began to seek my opinion and support with new product prototypes, and my bosses appreciated how hard I worked. I dared to hope that one day people would look at me and see someone great.

Chapter 6

God's Timing

*He who finds a wife finds a good thing
and obtains favor from the Lord.*
Proverbs 18:22

In 1992, I was twenty-six years old and trying to get my life on track. I went to church two or three times a month, usually at the 5:00 p.m. Mass at St. Patrick Church. It was the same church my family had always attended and was associated with my first five years of school. I sat in the same pew every week, as most people do. I'd like to say that I experienced inspiration and awe every time, but it was not quite that way. Rather, I found that the message usually didn't resonate with me, and the service structure was not well-suited to someone with an extremely limited attention span. To be honest, most of the time, I took in absolutely nothing. I was always glad that there wasn't a test at the end of the service because I would certainly have failed it, just like I'd so often failed in school.

One Saturday at Mass, I noticed one young woman about my age or a little younger sitting a few pews in front of me. She was definitely pretty, was attentive, and appeared devoted. I was intrigued. I went back to the same Mass the following week and every week or every other week after that for a few months and was glad to see her there more often than not. Staring at the back of her head week after week made it even more difficult for me to focus on the sermon, but at least it kept me coming back.

I finally worked up the courage to talk to her, and after Mass one day, I asked if she would go out with me to get something to eat. She politely replied that she was sorry, but she had a date that night and had to leave right away. There was an uncomfortable moment of silence between us before we awkwardly said goodbye to each other. I'll never forget walking back to my car stinging from her rejection, once again trying to understand why God didn't ever seem to take it easy on me and let things work out the way I wanted them to—even with a girl from church.

Of course, being turned down was never easy. I didn't usually ask a woman out if I hadn't met her before. I preferred instead to ask someone for a date only if I already knew her a bit. This way, I could consider whether or not the girl was likely interested enough in me to risk making my move. If the situation seemed promising, I tried to casually slide my request into the conversation as if it was no big deal. That way, if she said no, I'd just move on as if it wasn't a big deal.

In this case, though, I'd not had a chance to talk with the woman first, so I had to take the chance. After she said no, I stopped going to church—at least on Saturday evenings. I didn't stop going to bars, though, and it wasn't long before I was able to employ my preferred method of asking for a date at a spot I frequented in nearby Oshkosh, a larger city only twenty-five miles from my home. The woman I met there one night was pretty and seemed kind, but she was already a mom of three, including a baby. Even though I liked her, I wasn't sure this was a level of commitment I was ready to accept. The fact that she was technically still married was also a little bothersome, but I talked myself out of any great concern about it. *After all, they were separated,* I reasoned.

One night a short while after we'd had a few dates, the woman and I went to a bar where she and her friends liked to hang out. As we were getting ready to go, she discreetly pointed out the window to some men standing near my car. "That's my husband," she said. I took a glance and noticed a small group of men standing around as if they were waiting for something—or someone. Apparently, her husband had some friends with him, and they all looked pretty tough. Then the girl warned me that

God's Timing

her husband wouldn't hesitate to seriously hurt anyone who seemed to be accompanying her, and his buddies would be quick to reinforce his message. I was suddenly a little sick with anxiety. *Maybe we could just wait them out,* I thought. The night was quickly winding down, however, and the barkeeper had his own agenda. He soon announced that it was closing time and made it clear that we needed to leave. Almost all the other patrons had left by then, so there was no hope we could exit the place undetected in a crowd. Instead, we'd have to walk out of the building together, yet very alone.

All of a sudden, a police car pulled up behind the woman's husband and his companions. It pulled to a stop behind them in the parking lot, and an officer got out. I could hardly believe my eyes. When the officer began to converse with the group, we hustled to my car, jumped in, and zipped away. I raced straight to her house, where she quickly got out and ran to the door. Once I saw she was safely inside, I sped away again, thankful for the darkness and the intervention of a well-timed police officer.

At the time, I attributed this near-miraculous event to a stroke of good luck, but in my later years, I considered it wasn't likely luck at all—it was God's protection and guiding hand. He didn't want me to contribute in any way to the breaking of another's marriage covenant. At the time, I only recognized the threat of punishment from her husband, but later on, it was clear that being with a married woman would have also greatly displeased God. I'm glad He helped me recognize this before I could do any more damage to our relationship—and before the woman's husband could do any damage to me. As I drove away from the woman's home that fateful night, I knew I'd never see her again.

After breaking up with the woman, I took a little time off from dating and the bar scene, but soon another kind of difficulty came into my life. One night when I was alone in my apartment, I had just completed my favorite meal: a large cheesy, saucy, extra-sausage pizza. When I got out of my chair to get another large glass of milk from the refrigerator, I suddenly felt a strange sensation in my abdomen, as if some part of my stomach had just snapped like a rubber band. I doubled over in pain, wobbled to my bed, and collapsed upon it. For several hours, I laid there in discomfort, extremely worried and confused about what had happened. Eventually, I fell asleep, but the next morning I awoke to the same intense pain I'd felt the night before.

The discomfort slowly subsided throughout the next few days, but it seemed wise for me to be very careful about what I ate for a while. Eventually, I went back to eating most foods, but I felt like I should avoid large amounts of cheese and other dairy products. I didn't even have pizza again for many months. I'd definitely given it a lot of thought. Still, I'd not been able to determine what had made my stomach snap and then hurt so badly, and I worried that it would happen again. Maybe it would be even more severe the next time.

Even though my stomach seemed to heal from the stabbing pain I'd initially felt, I now occasionally noticed digestive issues I'd not had before: large amounts of gas, back pain, stomach aches, and diarrhea. Sometimes I'd have just one issue at a time, and at other times, I'd experience all of them together. After several uncomfortable episodes, I finally decided to see a doctor.

The general practitioner I saw didn't know what had caused my problems, so he sent me to a specialist. The specialist ordered some tests. Then, although he also couldn't identify what might have caused the snapping sensation or the intense pain, he prescribed some pills that he said could help my stomach pain. I was glad to have pills to take away the pain. By the time I finished the bottle, I felt better and was pleased to be over that hurdle—or so I thought.

Now my stomach felt better, but I began to notice other problems with my health. One of my biggest new concerns was the onset of dizzy spells—some of which were pretty severe. The first intense spell occurred at work while I was preparing to run a machine. I was standing behind it when I began to feel lightheaded. As the dizziness swiftly intensified, I grabbed onto one of the machine's bars to wait it out. Eventually, it passed, and I continued with my work. I had a few more dizzy spells that day and at least one almost every day after that for several weeks. I tried to believe that the dizziness was likely caused by a virus or some other benign condition, but it quickly became clear there was more to them than that.

Once again, I made an appointment with the general practitioner, and once again, he referred me to a specialist who ordered some tests. I was asked to return about a week later to hear the results. At this appointment, the specialist told me that the tests didn't reveal anything unusual and therefore didn't have much to suggest. He told me that it was possible that my dizziness was due to a condition called Meniere's Disease—an inner ear disorder characterized by vertigo, ear congestion, hearing loss, and ringing in the ears. Since I had some of those symptoms, it seemed like this could be the problem. Unfortunately, the specialist informed me that there weren't any medications to help with Meniere's Disease, although some people found relief by eliminating salt from their diet. Overall, people with Meniere's Disease just had to live with the symptoms. Since I'd imagined that my issue might be a brain tumor or other serious issue, I probably should have been relieved by what I had been told. The thought, however, of living the rest of my life with severe dizzy spells and diet restrictions was discouraging.

In the following months, I did my best to avoid salt, but it was difficult. I took low or no-salt options in my lunch to work, but I sure did miss my ham and cheese sandwiches and subs. I noticed that avoiding caffeine and alcohol also helped to moderately reduce the number and severity of my dizzy spells. I didn't typically drink coffee or soda, though, so this only helped a little. When the weekends came around, I continued to enjoy a beer or two with my friends while trying to ignore the fact that my body never reacted well to it and that I really should avoid that, too. In addition to contributing to the dizzy spells, the hangovers I experienced after drinking it were massive. I'd have incredible headaches, flu-like symptoms, and extreme fatigue, often for two days or more. Ironically, it still took quite a while to convince me that this was not in my best interest because sometimes the reaction was less extreme or even nonexistent.

It wasn't so much that it was hard for me to give up drinking alcohol, but rather that I really enjoyed the environment of the bar. I enjoyed socializing with my friends, playing darts and pool, and meeting girls. That was the case on one Friday evening when a few friends and I headed out to some of our favorite local bars. We stuck together for the early part of the night, but eventually, my friends went their own way, leaving me sitting alone amongst the noisy Friday night crowd. A beautiful girl, with what appeared to be a few of her friends, was standing next to me. As people moved through the crowd, she was often nudged close to me, during which we exchanged a few comments. After a few such occasions, we began a lengthier conversation, and before I knew it, we'd been talking for about half an hour. Her name was Mary. When her friends urged her to go with them across the street to another bar, we said goodbye, but before she left, she suggested that I join them there.

I wanted to play it cool, so I hung out at the original bar for a while, then followed her across the street a short time later. I "bumped into her" there and we picked up the conversation once again. At Bar Time, I asked Mary for her phone number and was thrilled that she agreed to share it with me! I fought off the usual rush of feelings that tried to trick me into falling instantly for a girl. By Wednesday of the next week, though, I was still convinced I wanted to get to know her better, so I gave her a call. I asked if she'd like to go out for some pizza, then to my nephew's high school football game on the coming Friday night. She agreed, so it was a date! By this time in my life, I'd been disappointed by a date or two, so I tried not to get my hopes up.

One date turned into two, then three, and eventually, we were spending most of our free time together. I could tell she liked me right away. Nevertheless, I was hesitant to allow myself to fall in love with her, even though she was smart, beautiful, and well-educated. A few years earlier, she would have been everything I could have hoped for, yet my anxiety about the pain I'd experience if she chose to end the relationship was so strong that I couldn't allow myself to commit to her fully.

Two months later, we were still together and getting to know each other better. Ironically, she was a teacher at the same small Catholic school I'd attended as a child and thus went to Mass at the same church I'd been attending. One day, it dawned on us, at almost the exact same time, that she was the girl I'd asked out a year or so earlier. My excuse for not recognizing her was that I had mostly seen only the back of her head, and hers was that she hadn't really seen me much since I was usually sitting behind her. In addition, I'd recently started wearing contact lenses instead of glasses, and she'd changed her hairstyle from one that was long and curly to one that was quite short and much straighter. It was hard to believe that this could be true, but there was no doubt that it was. The situation was so strange that I could only attribute it to

God's intervention, which significantly calmed my nerves about becoming involved with her.

During this time, Mary invited me to go along with her to visit her parents and some of her siblings. Situations like this are always uncomfortable because of how important it is to impress the family of the girl you are with, and this one turned out to be even more awkward than usual. Although the day started out fine, I quickly began to feel small and insignificant amongst her family. They were all polite and pleasant, but they were also very well-spoken and highly educated. Their conversation centered around their college experiences and professional lives. Since I'd barely finished high school and couldn't read or write very well, I felt like a misfit and certainly didn't feel worthy of dating one of them. Nonetheless, I knew there were a few things working in my favor: I was polite, didn't swear, knew a lot about sports, and liked playing golf, which was something that at least a few of them also enjoyed. In addition, I was up on the latest political news, and my views in this regard seemed to match those of the rest of the family. Outside of this, though, I felt like an outsider. I couldn't help but envy this crowd of people with a college education instead of just a high school diploma and a career instead of just a job. It is hard to say if her family was disappointed in me or if I simply projected that feeling upon myself, but it sure made that gathering a difficult one.

Because I worked the second shift and Mary worked almost opposite hours, it was hard to spend time together during the week. I would typically call her during my supper break and then stop by on my way home from work to visit for an hour or two. It wasn't the most convenient arrangement—especially for Mary—but young love is pretty resilient, so it didn't feel too difficult for either of us. On the weekend, we'd go to a bar to have a few drinks, eat pizza and watch a football game, or go out to eat and watch a movie. Mary enjoyed my company, and I enjoyed hers, even if we were just snuggled on the couch together watching something on TV in my little apartment.

I soon discovered that this was the first long-term relationship for Mary, so our relationship was something that she took pretty seriously. She claims she knew from the start that she wanted to marry me and was waiting for me to realize that I wanted the same. I'd made it clear early on that I had been hurt pretty deeply after previous breakups, and I wasn't going to put myself in that position again. So, she had a bit of an uphill climb, but she persisted. She delivered cards and treats to my mailbox on her way to school several times a week and made sure I knew she was interested in being with me. I was very much interested in being with her, too, but I wasn't very interested in having my heart broken again.

By the time we had been together for several months, I knew I had fallen in love, and it was so very different from my last serious relationship. This time, I hadn't hidden anything from her. I didn't want to go through what I had in the past: falling in love with someone, then being dropped because I had been hiding the parts of myself that could scare her away. She knew all my shortcomings: my inability to read well, my struggle with spelling, my blue-collar job, and even bits and pieces of my health issues. Instead of feeling insecure, I felt safe with her. She was never critical or judgmental; instead, she was understanding and encouraging. She was just what I needed. I started to hope I was just what she needed, too.

After dating for about four months, I had really started to feel comfortable with her. I not only loved her, but I trusted her and was ready for us to make more of a commitment to each other. I started to drop some hints to see how she might react. Her eager responses were positive and enthusiastic, and we soon began talking about looking for a ring and becoming engaged. One Saturday, a few weeks later, I asked Mary if she would come with me to the store. From the look on her face, she knew what I was thinking. We bounded down the narrow stairway that led out of my apartment building and into my car. Five minutes later, we were in the jewelry store. "We're looking for a ring," we told the attendant.

I had been to the jewelers a few times before just to take a look at what was available. I knew how beautiful diamond rings were and how expensive they were. Although I didn't make a lot of money, this was important. I told her to pick out whatever ring she desired as we began to look through the glass at the sparkling diamonds below. She browsed for a few minutes and then slowly moved toward the outer edge of the collection. She was drawn not to the large shiny jewels but to the small, simple ones. I have to admit I was a little disappointed. She didn't want something big or fancy but instead preferred a ring that was small and delicate. I wanted her to have something she could show off to my friends, but as is her way, she wanted something more understated, more suited to her personality.

After only a few minutes, I could tell I wasn't going to persuade her otherwise—and, remembering how I had insisted that she pick the ring of her choice, I stepped closer to look at her final choices with her. The attendant took out a few samples for us to study before Mary selected the one that she liked the best. I joked it was good to know what kind of ring she liked if ever I might need to know something like that (wink, wink).

Several weeks later, we were watching TV in my apartment when I received a phone call. I had ordered the ring Mary had chosen almost right after she had picked it out, and the jeweler was calling to let me know it was ready to be picked up. I toyed with the idea of telling Mary a story of some kind so I could sneak down to the store to get it without her knowing, but I was too excited to play games. I just told her we had to go downtown to get something. She looked at me, and I knew she knew. Still, she didn't say anything, even as we got into the car, drove it downtown, and parked on the road in front of the jewelry store. Leaving Mary in the car, I went in, paid for the ring, put it in my pocket, and hurried back to the car. We rode in silence back to my apartment, each of us contemplating the importance of what was to come. Almost as soon as we arrived back at my apartment, I went down on one knee and asked Mary to marry me. She instantly said, "Yes!"

We hugged and kissed and hugged and kissed some more. We had just cemented our future together and were so happy. Like most newly engaged couples, of course, neither of us realized the gravity of the situation. Young love is bubbly and exciting, but it is also fleeting. Mature love is very different. Mary and I had a lot to learn about ourselves and each other.

Our wedding date was set for just over a year later, so once we were engaged, there was a lot of time for planning. Most of the time, though, life continued on as it always had. At this point, of course, I'd already dealt with some health issues, but I didn't think of myself as sickly because, most of the time, I felt relatively okay. Unfortunately, I soon began to experience many new and unusual symptoms—all of which seemed to be unrelated. I spent a lot of time thinking about them, and when I began to explain them to my new fiancé, it became clear to both of us that I'd really been challenged with physical ailments since my childhood. I'd been hospitalized with an unexplained condition when I was just four years old and grew up with frequent ear infections, incredibly bloody noses, and ringing in my ears. I struggled with memory and attention issues in school from first grade through high school and began to have dizzy spells, food intolerances, stomach distress, and vision difficulties as a young adult—issues just kept popping up and piling on to each other.

At the time, my biggest health complaint was my stomach. I was having the same problems I'd experienced after my incident with the pizza. Mary thought the best thing would be to seek a specialist to help us determine what was going on. So I made an appointment with a gastroenterologist at the highly esteemed Marshfield Clinic in Marshfield, Wisconsin.

I think we both feared knowing more about my condition. Perhaps this is why it had taken me so long to set up an appointment. I know I was hoping that if I just avoided my pesky symptoms, they might just go away. I certainly didn't want to hear that I was suffering from any kind of terminal issue. I'd rather just die suddenly than have to face the emotional pain of hearing about it. Of course, there was always the possibility of a doctor telling me that if I had just come in two months earlier, something could have been done about whatever problem I had. The emotional part of being sick sure can be tough because our minds don't think rationally when it comes to matters out of our control, especially regarding life and death issues.

Since my appointment involved a colonoscopy, I fasted, did the appropriate cleaning out, and arrived at the clinic early on the day of the procedure. A few days later, I received a call from the doctor who told me that my abdominal discomfort was likely caused by a condition called ulcerative colitis. This chronic disease of the large intestines can cause feelings of fatigue, low energy, loss of appetite, abdominal pain, cramping, diarrhea, and bleeding. I had all of those things, so it seemed that he was right. Although it didn't explain the dizziness I'd now been experiencing for several years, I assumed that it was something separate altogether and that I'd just been lucky enough to have these conditions at once. I was surprised that neither of these diagnoses accounted for any of the ailments I'd experienced as a child, such as the incredible nosebleeds and frequent ear ringing. Since they'd mostly faded away over time, I figured they might always just be a mystery to me. At any rate, there wasn't much else to do but take the physician's advice. I was given a prescription for a drug called Sulfasalazine and told to watch what I ate.

I took the medicine every day and planned a colonoscopy every two years. My stomach started to improve, but not consistently. I would feel good for a couple of months, then bad for a few weeks, then better again. The dizzy spells, however, didn't seem to be letting up at all despite my low-salt diet. To complicate things, new and unusual symptoms seemed to come and go randomly. It seemed as if there was something still going on inside of me that hadn't been identified or treated.

Mary began to research my symptoms and discovered some interesting parallels with those present when one is experiencing food allergies. According to the information she'd uncovered, some people reacted to food not with throat swelling or hives but with dizziness, brain fog, or abdominal discomfort. So perhaps my condition was neither ulcerative colitis nor Meniere's disease, but food allergies. This food allergy concept seemed like something we needed to investigate further, and we were intrigued and excited by the hope this had sparked.

Chapter 7

For Better or for Worse

And not only this, but we also celebrate in our tribulations, knowing that tribulation brings about perseverance; and perseverance, proven character; and proven character, hope; and hope does not disappoint, because the love of God has been poured out within our hearts through the Holy Spirit who was given to us.
Romans 5:3-5

In our quest to get to the bottom of my health issues, we decided to see a renowned food allergist in Oshkosh, which is about thirty-five minutes from Ripon. I knew nothing about allergists at the time or what an allergist does to determine a person's allergies. If I did, I would have been a whole lot less enthused about the situation.

The clinic had scheduled a skin prick test. Once my name was called and my vitals were taken, the nurse had me remove my shirt. She then used a pen to mark dots in a pattern of about ten rows of five columns across my back. She also marked some from my upper arm down to my elbow. Next to each dot, she pricked my skin with a tool upon which she'd placed a drop of a common allergen. The plan was to see whether or not my skin would react to the allergen. I was told a reaction would show as a small bump, swelling, or minor area of itching at the site. I remember them saying "small" and "minor," but my reaction was definitely neither. Within minutes I had a back full of incredibly itchy and extremely uncomfortable bumps. I had an allergic reaction to almost everything for which I was tested.

When the doctor arrived to examine my skin after the skin prick test, he raised his eyebrows in surprise. He took a piece of paper, placed it against his clipboard, and drew a standard bell-shaped curve. "In a nutshell," he said, "Yours is a case that would be marked way over here," and he pointed to the far-right end of the diagram. I was stunned as he continued without so much as a shrug or a sympathetic grimace, coldly informing me that "There just isn't much that can be done about the situation." According to this doctor, taking pills or shots to alleviate any allergic reactions was pointless because they wouldn't make a big enough impact to be of much help. "The only thing that would really help," he said, "would be to avoid the items that might affect you."

I was discouraged. Was he kidding? I was apparently allergic to everything. How was I supposed to avoid *everything?* It was quickly apparent that the doctor didn't have any further advice for me and was soon out the door. I was more than a little dismayed that he'd responded with so little empathy and little to no help. As I gathered my things, I couldn't help but feel overwhelmed. How was I going to handle this? Moreover, what if things got worse over time? Mary and I discussed what we'd learned on the drive home and came to the conclusion that there wasn't much else to do other than to hope that a medical discovery would eventually be found that could help me.

Despite my depressing health outlook, our lives during that year weren't all doom and gloom. We were newly engaged, after all, and had a lot to look forward to. Mary was busy making plans, and I was busy supporting them. She knew what she wanted, and since I didn't feel strongly one way or the other, I practiced being a good listener and encourager.

If God cared at all about giving me a good life, it seemed like He was finally doing so. Mary was the selfless, generous, beautiful woman I had always wanted to marry. When I thought about how God had sent her to be my wife, I was hopeful it was a sign that He'd finally begun to care about me. Maybe He did have a plan for me. Maybe He even loved me.

For the time being, although my physical health wasn't great, it was at least stable. I avoided as much problematic food as I could and took medication for the ulcerative colitis. I still had digestive flare-ups, but they were less severe and less frequent. I was still having several severe dizzy spells but began to consider that they were more likely related to food allergies than caused by Meniere's Disease. Mary and I hoped we would find the answers we were looking for sooner rather than later, assuming that surely we'd meet a doctor or come across information about a unique condition at some point that would shed some light upon what was going on inside me.

Unfortunately, in the following months, my body slowly but surely became irritated by a growing number of foods. To add to the confusion, some bothered me one time but didn't seem to bother me another, and vice-versa. In addition, a certain food might be troublesome only if I had it more than once in close succession, but it wouldn't have a noticeable effect on me if I waited longer before eating it again.

It was about this time that I started to have problems with my neck. Occasionally, it was difficult for me to get my mind and muscles to work together to turn my head as I'd like. Once they did, my neck would often suddenly become tight and uncomfortable. At other times, my neck would stiffen immediately after or during a dizzy spell. Sometimes worrying about the possibility of a severe dizzy spell caused my neck muscles to tighten. On other occasions, my neck seemed to tighten for no other reason at all.

One Sunday, while I was waiting to receive Holy Communion at church, I had a severe dizzy spell. Of course, I became nervous, especially so because I was a long way from my pew—there wasn't much to grab onto except strangers to my front, back, and sides. Just being worried about passing out, of course, made my neck lock up. It took all of the concentration I could muster to take Holy Communion, turn the corner, then another, make it up the slightly inclined aisle, and turn again to make it along the pews back to my seat. This was the start of a whole new set of worries for me. I now began to have anxiety about passing out in full view of others, especially my colleagues at work and my friends on the golf course.

With our wedding day approaching, I began to worry about how I was going to be able to manage everything. There was probably no time when one is the focus of attention more than this. How in the world was I going to make it? I tried working on staying in the present: managing my condition moment by moment. Still, every day I was frustrated, confused, and angry that no medical specialists had been able to—or even seemed interested to—help me determine what was going on with me, how all of my physical symptoms might be related, and what the outcome of my struggles might be. How could it be that no physicians had ever heard of that with which I was dealing? How could it be that with all the research that is done in laboratories around the world, no one had ever encountered a situation like this anywhere? Was I really the only one with this condition? I was becoming increasingly frustrated.

The warmth of spring turned to the dry heat of summer, and before we knew it, our big day, June 18, had arrived. When I woke up that morning, I thought about how I once wondered if my wedding day would ever come. Then my thoughts immediately switched to my health. My excitement couldn't surpass my concern about whether I would make it through the ceremony. I had never liked the spotlight. In school, I don't think I ever raised my hand—even if I thought I was a hundred-percent sure of the answer (although I'm a hundred-percent sure I was never a hundred-percent sure of the answer). In meetings at work, my voice cracked when answering a simple question. I was always afraid of people laughing at me, so I knew it was just easier to avoid the spotlight. Today, though, I was going to be in the spotlight, and I had to somehow deal with it. It was one thing to do this while feeling healthy, but quite another to do so when you're not even sure you're going to physically be able to make it through something. I just didn't trust my body to do what I wanted it to do.

My mind began to obsess and play out negative scenarios over and over again.

I arrived at the church conflicted. I was definitely excited to be married to my lovely fiancé, but the day wasn't one I was happily anticipating because I was so worried that my body wasn't going to cooperate with my plans. I didn't want to embarrass myself or Mary by passing out or making some sort of scene while having a major dizzy spell. Of course, when my anxiety grew, my physical issues increased: my muscles tightened, making it difficult for my body to respond to my brain's commands. It took extreme concentration to get my eyes and head to move the way I wanted them to. I wished I could have put aside all my worries to enjoy this special day, but I just wanted it to be over.

Eventually, the church was filled with family members and friends, and the moment had arrived for me to make my entrance. I moved into place and tried to casually smile at our loved ones who were looking expectantly at me. My real focus, however, was upon the long, descending aisle ahead. The altar seemed so far away. I took a deep breath and then stepped one foot forward. Then the other. *Right. Left. Right. Left. Deep breath. Concentrate. Right. Left. Smile. Act nonchalant. Stand tall. Breathe. Look around. Smile. Right. Left. Breathe.*

I was thrilled when I finally arrived at the altar and let the weight of a thousand worries slide off my shoulders. I'd made it! I was right where I needed to be, and I was thrilled. I looked at my gorgeous bride and grinned. Some of that smile was meant for her, but honestly, most of it was in celebration that the hardest part of the day was over and that I'd made it through what had worried me for so long.

Throughout the Mass, my neck occasionally stiffened for a moment or two. Still, I was able to stave it off by forcing myself to take a deep, relaxing breath and trying hard to just focus on the moment. Finally, after considerable effort, we entered the latter half of the ceremony, and the light at the end of the tunnel got brighter and brighter. Was I really going to make it through this without incident? All I had to do was hang in there for a little while longer.

Soon the priest was giving his final blessing, signaling the end of the Mass. I could hardly contain my relief. I'd made it! The rest of the day was going to be not just a celebration of my marriage but a celebration that this major challenge was behind me. The rest of the day and into the night were filled with complete happiness. It was definitely the best day of my life.

We had planned a trip to The French Quarter in New Orleans to celebrate our wedding. I'd always wanted to go there because I've also always loved music—especially live bands like the ones we'd see there. Also, since Mary didn't have a preference about where to go, it seemed like the perfect choice. I'd only been out of the state of Wisconsin a few times before and had never even flown in a plane, so the honeymoon promised to be full of many exciting adventures for the new Mr. and Mrs. John Wagner.

Unfortunately, my life wasn't as carefree as it once had been because of my declining health, so going on vacation was more complicated than it otherwise would have been. I was living on a fairly restricted diet. I wasn't sure how my digestive tract would do when eating out all the time rather than eating what I'd prepared myself the way I knew my stomach would best tolerate the food. In addition, my recent appointment with the allergist highlighted how reactive I was to foods and the environment. It, therefore, wasn't a stretch to think I could have an allergic reaction to something I'd never tried before (like one of the seafoods so common in Louisiana) or to suddenly or possibly or even seriously react to something I'd ingested before without any problem. I'd had tingling lips or a numb tongue after eating a food in the past, so I knew a reaction of some severity was possible. I didn't know, however, how likely it was (or wasn't) that it could be life-threatening.

Thankfully, my anxiety about food turned out to be a bigger worry in my head than in my digestive tract. I cautiously tried a few new items, and each one turned out to be a delicious and safe choice. On our first night in New Orleans, Mary and I ordered a large serving of crawdads. They were served in a bowl, almost like popcorn, and they were delicious! Even better was the fact that my body seemed to accept them without any difficulty at all. I had several bowls of those delicious crawdads while we were in New Orleans, and it was definitely a treat every time!

Another meal I enjoyed was jambalaya. I ordered it without shrimp just to be safe and didn't even miss the little critters. It was wonderful! Throughout the whole trip, the only food-related reaction I had was a minor dizzy spell right after eating one of the meals.

The sun, on the other hand, took over where the food left off. We were so thankful to be where it was sunny and warm that we spent much of the afternoon in and beside the hotel swimming pool. We were watching for signs of sunburn, but it wasn't until we came back inside that we noticed how red my back and chest were. I took some ibuprofen as soon as I could to stop the burn from deepening, but it wasn't soon enough. I was fried! Skin tenderness was only the first of my problems from the sunburn: shivers, a headache, and overall body pain soon followed. The rest of the day, that night, and the following day were miserable.

The sunburn pain gradually subsided enough so we could get back to enjoying our experience. Maybe the music, excellent food, and interesting people around us helped speed the healing. The unique lifestyle and culture of The French Quarter were definitely a treat. The rest of the week passed quickly, and soon it was time for us to fly back home and begin our life together.

We returned to Wisconsin and our new apartment. It was a duplex, and we were fortunate enough to have the entire downstairs portion of the building to ourselves. It was newly remodeled, so it was modern, clean, and very comfortable. This nice living space, in addition to my recent move from second to first shift at my job, provided us with some blissful opportunities together despite my ever-present health challenges.

Chapter 8

And Baby Makes Three

*Behold, children are a gift of the Lord,
The fruit of the womb is a reward.*
Psalm 127:3

Life was wonderful for us as we settled into marriage with no additional, unexpected challenges. Mary and I worked normal hours, enjoyed our cozy new apartment, and adjusted well to living together. She was ready to start a family right away, but I wasn't as anxious. I wasn't opposed to the idea, but it wasn't a huge priority for me. We decided to leave it up to God.

As is so often the case when we initially tell God to take the lead, Mary quickly got tired of waiting. She began to talk about whether or not we should see a specialist to make sure everything was working correctly for both of us since it had been nearly six months, and she hadn't yet become pregnant. Then one Saturday morning in early February, Mary walked over to me in the living room. I was probably watching a game of some kind on TV and hadn't noticed that she'd just exited the bathroom with a curious smirk on her face.

Mary smiled, sat beside me on the couch, and handed me a pregnancy test strip without saying much at all. Of course, I had no idea how to read the test, but I knew enough to speculate that her smiling and handing it to me probably meant she was happy about what she'd seen. Yup. We were about to become Mom and Dad to some little, beautiful baby.

"Are you sure?" I double-checked. "Maybe this thing is faulty?"

Mary shrugged in a way that said, "I'm pretty sure!" Still, she obliged me and suggested we drive to the store to get another one of a different brand. The result was the same.

By now, the excitement was starting to grow. Our imaginations began to run away with the thoughts and dreams of an incredible new adventure with a precious little addition to our family—a part of both of us to reflect our love and joy in the home. We decided to keep quiet about the news for a while, which was difficult because we were so very excited. When just the two of us were together, it was almost impossible to stop the "I wonders" and "I can't waits" that were flooding our brains.

While we were joyful and proud, we were also anxious about what was to come. One of our thoughts was about how well the apartment would suit our expanding family, and we began to consider how nice it would be to raise our child (and future children) in a home of our own. So we began to peruse home listings in the newspaper and for sale signs on front lawns, then set up tours through a few local houses.

One day, Mary noticed an ad in the paper showing a ranch home on a cul-de-sac in a wonderful part of town. It seemed so good that it would be sold quickly, so Mary set up an appointment to view it right away. One step into the house was all it took to recognize that this was the place for us. It was well-built and well cared for. It had three bedrooms, two bathrooms, a large kitchen, and a living room. It had a fireplace, a full basement, a double garage, and a beautiful backyard. Best of all, the price was lower than we'd expected. We put in an offer that same day, and almost without delay, the house was ours! At one point, I recall considering that not too long ago, I was sitting alone in my small apartment, wondering why God had allowed me to be abandoned by a woman I was sure was the only one that could make me happy. Then, the next thing I knew, I was married to a woman who was perfect for me, expecting a beautiful baby and signing the papers to our own home. *How did all of this happen?*

I thought. *Why had it been so hard for me to trust God's plans for me?*

On Friday, September 15, 1995, Mary worked all day. Although the baby was two days overdue, she didn't think anything of the barely-discernible physical sensations she'd been experiencing. Perhaps since this was her first pregnancy, she didn't realize that she'd actually been in labor for most of the day! When she arrived home from work, she lay down on the couch to relax as we talked about our day and made plans for the evening. We considered going to the mall to walk around and do some window shopping, but when she nonchalantly mentioned that she didn't feel "right," I knew we needed to contact the doctor so she could explain her symptoms to him. It took a while to convince her to do so because she was pretty sure that whatever was going on didn't have anything to do with the baby. Nevertheless, Mary eventually agreed just to be safe. It took only a minute or two for the doctor to direct her to the hospital for an examination.

At the hospital, she put on the gown she was given, then waited for the nurse to examine her. It didn't take long before it was proclaimed that Mary was, without a doubt, in labor. We looked at each other, shocked but excited. The nurse suggested that walking would continue to move the process along, so that's what we did. Sure enough, walking began to accelerate things: the baby's positioning as well as the discomfort. Mary wanted to give birth without medication, which meant every advancement toward the goal required increased pain. I quickly discovered my input wasn't needed or appreciated, so I tried to be as helpful as possible by just standing nearby—not touching anything, saying anything, or even breathing in any way that could be construed as irritating to her.

The duration of the labor at the hospital was pretty quick, considering that it had been occurring for most of the day, and it wasn't long before I was holding our new baby girl in my arms. I know it sounds trite, but except for Mary, Julia was the prettiest thing I'd ever seen. I was mesmerized by her sweet little face and instantly felt a depth of love that I'd never before experienced.

Our family's first hours together were surreal. Once Julia's needs had been addressed, she'd had her first feeding, and we'd done a fair amount of oohing and aahing at the blessing we'd received, it was time to turn down the lights and rest for a bit. Perhaps my sleeplessness during that time was the result of the stiff vinyl chair I had been given for a bed, but it was more likely because of my desire to sneak just one more peek at the beautiful angel wrapped in pink who was peeping contentedly in the bassinet beside Mary. In the dark, nurses occasionally snuck in quietly to check on my girls, and as the new day dawned, their visits became more frequent. We were so thankful for their attentiveness, wisdom, and care. They treated us as if we were the most important concern in the world, thoroughly explaining everything that needed to be done. I would typically be groggy and grouchy after only a few hours of low-quality sleep. On that day, though, I couldn't have been more awake and joyful!

On Day Two, it was time for us to leave the hospital to do The Parenting Thing all by ourselves. Although I was a little anxious, I was mostly curious. What would fatherhood be like with a newborn, then a toddler, then an older child, a teen, and even an adult? I wished I could see into the future to know what Julia would be like during all of those stages and to know more about the adventures we'd have together.

Mary and Julia were discharged from the hospital during the mid-morning. Mary's parents brought some lunch and spent some time visiting, but it wasn't long before it was just the three of us. We brought Julia's bassinet out into the living room and carefully laid her in it after she'd fallen asleep in Mary's arms. She took up such a small part of it! God's tiny yet fully human creation with ten perfect little fingers and toes and her earlobes and nose was such an amazing gift.

Since Julia was asleep, it seemed logical for me to get on with my typical weekend pastime: golf. I reasoned that even though our baby's first day at home was significant, it was just the first of many more days I could spend with Julia in my lifetime. Mary didn't stop me as I made plans to meet up with my buddies, and even if she had, it wouldn't have made much difference at that point in my life. I adored my wife, of course, and would have taken a bullet for either her or Julia. Honestly, though, I was probably more selfish than I'd like to admit.

I think I was so wrapped up in myself because I was angry about all the challenges I'd had to face in my life so far. I'd gone through a very difficult childhood and was now dealing with physical ailments that were making my young adulthood pretty uncomfortable, too. I told myself that life owed me happiness, and since golf made me happy, I should be allowed to golf whenever I was able. Even a newborn baby I loved wasn't going to get in the way of that.

Mary was allowed six weeks of maternity leave, and although she was home all day, she didn't consider it anything like a vacation. From my point of view, however, I was still working full-time and not feeling very well most days. Therefore, it was only fair for Mary to be the one to get up in the middle of the night to take care of the baby so I could get the sleep I needed to make it through the next day at work. Mary seemed to understand and took the challenge without much dissent. Those six weeks passed quickly, though, and when Mary went back to work, I knew it was time for me to pick up some more of the responsibilities. Still, when Julia fussed in the middle of the night, I typically pretended not to notice.

I'd heard some rumors (which may have originated with Mary) that dads in some households got up at night to bring the baby to the mom at feeding time or to keep her company while she was up—at least once in a while. Even if this was true, I felt it wasn't a fair proposal because most guys didn't need as much sleep as I did to feel well-rested. In addition, since I worked around hot ovens and sharp knives every day, it was critical for me to be fully alert at all times. Grogginess that clouded my thinking or slowed my reactions could have serious consequences. As you might imagine, Mary had a different opinion about the situation.

Thankfully, just as it was getting desperately tense between us, Julia began to sleep through the night. Aside from occasional nighttime wakeups, Mary and I evenly shared most of the child-rearing and household responsibilities and got along well together, despite the demands in our lives. Things were looking up again.

When Julia was about a year old, we discovered Mary was pregnant again. This was definitely a surprise. Although we were thrilled, we were also nervous about the arrival of another newborn without having yet fully recovered from the first. To add fuel to the fire, this was about the same time that my allergies and intolerances once again started to get out of hand. I had even more issues now than when I visited the allergist several years before, and since it had been a while, we wondered if something new had been discovered and/or if a different allergist might have a different approach that could help me. We were still convinced that I wasn't a completely unique case and that even if my situation was more complex than most, there had to be others like me who they'd been able to help. So we made an appointment, and I began to feel excited about the possibility of finding some relief.

Unfortunately, my optimism was short-lived. After more tests and more money, we were given a smile, a shrug, and another bunch of the same kind of bad news from this second allergist. Apparently, there was still nothing that could be done to help me. I was incredibly annoyed and disheartened, but Mary continued to be optimistic and right away began searching for someone else who might be able to help me. She soon heard about a clinic called Allergy Associates of LaCrosse, which was located in a city only three hours from our home.

We were excited to find these well-respected specialists so close to home but were concerned about the cost of an appointment at this clinic. It didn't bother us that they used experimental techniques, but apparently it bothered our health insurance company because they refused to cover the cost of any of their treatments. Since our combined income at that time didn't allow us the luxury of having a lot of money left over after the bills were paid, we were conflicted about what to do. Eventually, we didn't feel like we had any options other than taking this chance.

The day before my appointment, we left Ripon for LaCrosse and checked into a hotel for the night. The next morning, we drove to the clinic. It took us a while to locate the building because it was tucked into an old building in a quiet part of town. We checked in and found a seat in a small, well-worn waiting room. My name was called after a short wait, so I followed the nurse to a small room where my vitals were taken. I was then asked to take my shirt off so I could be given a skin prick test and a few drops of something under my tongue. The nurse told me she'd return in about thirty minutes to evaluate my symptoms. When she came back, she looked at the reactions on my skin, asked me a few questions, wrote some notes, and then led me to another room to wait for the doctor. When it was finally time for me to meet with him, I wasn't surprised when he confirmed once again that I was allergic to many, many things and was definitely taken aback when the world-renowned doctor told me I was one of the hardest cases he'd ever seen. He had some ideas about how to proceed but was uncertain about whether or not his treatment would be helpful.

The doctor told me that the most significant allergic response my body had shown was to dust mites, so that was what he would focus on. The clinic would mix up a solution that I would take under my tongue a few times a day to lessen my reaction to them. He also gave me an informational pamphlet and a thin catalog filled with items we could purchase for our home that could help in other ways. Only time would tell if these magic drops would be the answer we were seeking. We allowed ourselves a glimmer of hope as we left the clinic that day.

By that time, I knew I was lactose intolerant. Unfortunately, I really loved dairy products and had a hard time avoiding them altogether. One day I woke up to legs that were itching like crazy. While I was scratching them, I noticed several small, painful nodules on my calves and ankles. I waited a few days, but the bumps didn't decrease in size, so I thought it would be a good idea to have someone take a look at the situation. This should have been an easy phone call to one of the local clinics. Still, because I'd seen so many physicians with so many unusual symptoms, I feared that I'd left most of them with the impression that I was just a hypochondriac who had nothing better to do with my time than to make things up for them to treat. I didn't want to have to face them again with yet another crazy situation. Also, since they hadn't helped me when I'd seen them previously, I didn't feel like it was worth it to give them another try.

Mary did some research and found an osteopathic physician that visited one of the local clinics once a week. I didn't know anything about osteopathic medicine at that time but was encouraged to try it when I learned that it involved a more holistic approach to healing than what might be used by the more traditional medical doctor. This might be just what I needed for this problem, and if I was lucky, perhaps the doctor would have insights that would help me with some of my other conditions as well. So I made an appointment and began to hope once again that this visit would lead to some answers.

When we arrived at the clinic, the physician took a quick look at my legs before naming the swollen nodules *erythema nodosum*. We were excited that the doctor was actually able to name the situation—and so quickly. Our enthusiasm dampened, however, when he told us that this was just a general term for a condition involving nodules—kind of like when someone says they have a rash. It's not a specific diagnosis but instead a very broad definition of a situation. According to the doctor, *erythema nodosum* is the development of tender red lumps under the skin on the shins or calves. Like a rash, its cause is often unknown. Essentially, we were back to Square One.

As was so often the case at my medical appointments, the doctor couldn't identify what had caused the bumps but told us that they'd eventually diminish on their own. Hence, they weren't something we needed to worry about too much. We left the clinic that day like we had so many times before: with less money in our pockets and just as much confusion in our brains. Thankfully, the bumps did go down after a week or so, but they also returned. Then they went away again and then came back. The situation repeated itself again and again. Each time they came and went, they left a permanent bruise or scar in their place.

Somewhere along the way, I began to wonder if the dairy products I'd been enjoying might be bothering more than just my intestines; if they might also be causing the nodules to develop. My hypothesis was proven true when I truly avoided dairy products for several weeks and noticed not only that the nodules went away but also that they didn't return. Sadly, that was the end of dairy altogether for me.

As my physical well-being continued to be challenged, so too was my mental health. I kept telling myself that I just had to be tough: to pick up the ball and finish the play—no matter what, like my mom had said to me so many years ago. It was really starting to wear me down.

So when Mary surprised me that day with the news that she was pregnant with our second child, I was thrilled! Still, almost immediately, I was also extremely anxious. We already had a little one at home who required a lot of time and energy, and I just didn't know if I could do everything that was expected of me for her, for Mary, and for our next child. I wanted to participate fully in my children's lives, not just now but for many years in the future, and was uncertain that I'd be able to do so with all the discomfort I was currently experiencing. I knew it was possible that even if I could ignore my present-day aches and pains, I may not be able to do so when I—and my children—were older.

May 23, 1997, might have started out as a regular day, but its end was far from ordinary. It was the date that our second child joined the family. That Friday morning, Mary got ready for work just as usual and planned to stop for a quick exam before school since she was so close to her due date. Ironically, she was closer to her due date than she knew because, after his brief examination, the doctor announced that today would be the day. A nurse settled Mary into one of the maternity rooms and started making preparations for the birth of a baby while Mary called me at work to let me know of the change in plans.

Mary remembered all too well what it had felt like to give birth without any medication, and although she loved the theory, she wasn't too fond of the reality. This time around, she planned to ask for relief when the pain rolled in. Unfortunately, even though her basic needs were well met by the nursing staff, the anesthesiologist with the long needle was not to be found. She waited and waited and tried to be tough and pleasant. She kind of drew into herself, literally gritted her teeth, and silently dealt with the excruciating pain. Finally, after several hours of waiting, the anesthesiologist arrived and administered the medication. It didn't take long for it to take effect, and soon Mary was smiling and at ease. We were both so excited to meet this new little one!

Our first view of Joseph showed that he was perfect in every way. He even had a neat side part in his hair. I was so excited to see him and hold him. I had amazing hopes and dreams for him and felt such immense pleasure as I considered my growing family. Since Baby Joe arrived during the day, we had more time with him before turning the lights down for the night. As with Julia, I settled in on the vinyl hospital chair, where once again, I slept very little and couldn't help but frequently peek over at Mary and the baby. Eventually, it was Saturday morning, and everyone knew what happened on Saturday: golf, of course!

Chapter 9

The Breaking Point

Therefore, since Christ has suffered in the flesh, arm yourselves also with the same purpose, because the one who has]suffered in the flesh has ceased from sin, so as to live the rest of the time in the flesh no longer for human lusts, but for the will of God.
1 Peter 4:1-2

I know most people spend the first days of a birth with their wife and new baby in the hospital, but by gosh, everybody knew I played golf on Saturdays! It was my very limited chance to spend some time with the guys. *After all, I never go out drinking,* I thought, trying to justify my actions. *I hardly ever play cards, either. So golf it is. Besides, you know how short the summers are in Wisconsin? Real short!* So while Mary and Baby Joe were resting and getting acquainted in the hospital, I headed out to play a round of golf.

If I'd been selfish with Child Number One, I was clearly even more so with Child Number Two. My reasoning seemed solid at the time, though: Mary and Joe would both just be lying around resting until the doctor released them. At that point, they would simply need to get in the car and drive the mile or so home. Moreover, since Mary was an experienced mom, she wouldn't need my advice about anything. Also, despite what she had just been through, she didn't seem physically challenged in any way.

After all, I figured, *she'd already been in and out of the hospital bed several times and moving around the room as if nothing extraordinary had just occurred. So it really won't be a big deal for me to be gone for a few hours.*

Mary still smirks a bit when she reminds me about how incredulous the hospital staff was when Mary packed up her things, put baby Joseph in the car seat, and discharged herself later that day. One of them even asked Mary if she was really okay driving herself home. Mary took it in stride, of course, acting like it didn't bother her that she was doing this by herself. I know, though, it must not have just *looked* weird—I know it felt weird to her, too.

I knew at the time that my actions that day were selfish, but I was so desperately seeking relief from the overwhelming and continual discomfort and dissatisfaction that filled my life. It wasn't fair that I continually had to say no to so much of life for reasons that were out of my control. No, you can't have a beer with your friends after work on Friday night. No, you can't have a piece of cake on your daughter's birthday. No, you can't have milk or bread or fruit or even most vegetables. No, you can't even have a day without a neck ache or headache or chest pain or vision problems or stomach distress, or some other unusual, uncomfortable issue. Also, no, you can't work in a job you'd really enjoy because you can't read or write well enough to go to school to do it, nor can you focus long enough to learn what would be taught there anyway. This life of mine was a big rip-off, so I was going to take what I wanted when I could get it—even if it meant that someone else had to give up something so I could do so.

Mary took care of Baby Jo Jo just like she had taken care of Julia. She again had six weeks of maternity leave and then returned to teaching. Once she was back to teaching and still getting up in the middle of the night, I felt bad for her. Still, there seemed to be very little I could do to help with those late-night/early-morning tasks. I was just so tired each day as it was—I believed there was no way I could have spared even a few minutes of sleep.

The second time around, though, was a lot harder on Mary. Taking care of a two-year-old and a baby meant things were often very hectic. There really was no end in sight to the stress and demands upon her.

Even so, I reasoned, *I'm pretty stressed, too, dealing with the relentless demands of my own uncooperative body*. Although during the summer months I always felt better, I was still far from well even then. The challenges I faced caused me to move through most days with gritted teeth. As a result, life wasn't very pleasant for me and, by default, not very satisfying for Mary, either. Both of us spent most of our time counting down to the weekend when Mary hoped to get some extra rest, and I got the chance to do some golfing. Unfortunately, with two young children at home, our visions weren't very compatible. Before and after golf, I hadn't much energy for anything else, and Mary was always on call to take care of family errands and meet the kids' needs. During the winter months, it was even worse. I wasn't going to play golf, but because I felt so crummy, I wasn't much help around the home, either.

I don't really know why golf was so rewarding for me, but I'm sure it had a lot to do with the camaraderie of spending time with my friends. Since I took up the game right after high school, I'd come to relish the challenge of a good game of golf on a beautiful summer day, topped off with conversation and a few drinks at the bar afterward. Although I could no longer drink alcohol or even soda because of its negative impact on my body, the experience still had some of the luster I'd come to expect. I wasn't completely unaware or unconcerned with Mary's needs while I was away. I always made sure I was home within a reasonable amount of time—usually six hours or so from the time I had left. Still, I didn't fully recognize—I probably didn't want to, to be honest—how hard my absence was on Mary while I was gone. She felt trapped at home with all of the responsibilities while I was out and about without any. This, in addition to her own fatigue, led to many conflicts over the years. I rationalized, of course, that this was Mary's fault. *She's probably just jealous. I have something I really enjoy and good friends to do it with, I told myself*. The problem, however, was deeper than that and involved misunderstanding between both of us. Mary thought I was being selfish for leaving her alone with all of the chores, and I thought that she was selfish for wanting to take my fun away. Neither of us saw the other's point of view, and after enough of these situations, we mostly stopped trying.

When the golf season ended, the stress between Mary and I should have dissipated. Since this was September, though, and was the time when Mary began planning for a new school year, it was a busy and anxious time for her. It was also the season when my airborne allergies started to really kick in. This stressed my body, which intensified the food-related issues I typically experienced. Ultimately, then, there was still plenty of tension in our home.

During the fall, Mary worked long and hard at school and came home to work long and hard here, too. I tried to do the same by ignoring my fatigue, allergies, and other physical discomforts. We were both comforted with the knowledge that once the new school year was underway, Mary would be able to relax just a bit there. Similarly, when the weather became colder and the ground froze, my allergies would loosen their grip on me. There seemed to be nothing else to do but hang on and hope we'd make it.

When December finally arrived, the ragweed pollen was no longer in the air. Hence, I had more energy relief from its symptoms and better overall health because my body wasn't as stressed. Moreover, Mary had settled into the school year routine a bit, so even though she was busy, she had this added comfort. In addition, the atmosphere at home was boosted by our lightened loads and the upcoming Christmas holiday—such an enchanting time with little ones brought much happiness.

One of our new family traditions included finding the perfect Christmas tree and adorning it with lights and ornaments in our living room. This was the case in 1999. About two weeks before Christmas, I began to experience flu symptoms of a sore throat, earache, headache, and generally thick feeling in my head that I had come to refer to as brain fog. Plus, I ached everywhere! All I could think of was sleep, and although I tried to be helpful, I had almost no strength or energy. I couldn't believe that at this time, which was supposed to be happy and relatively carefree, I was, once again, drastically sick.

Having heard this so many times before, Mary started losing her patience and compassion toward me. She began questioning whether it could really be true that I was sick and, therefore, unable to help out at home once again. One particularly frustrating day, after I told her I was going to lie down and watch TV for a while in the bedroom because I wasn't feeling well, she let it out. "Are you kidding me? You're sick again? No one in the world is sick as often as you are!" In exasperation, she continued. "John, you need to just toughen up and deal with this like a man! I'm so tired of living like this!"

What Mary didn't realize was that I was more tired of living like this than she was and that I was dealing with things as well as I could. The last thing I wanted was for anyone—especially Mary—to think I wasn't tough enough. I tried my best to pick up the ball and finish the play every single day. It was so hard, though, because the discomfort didn't ever seem to end.

I continued to be violently sick that year until about New Year's Day, when suddenly, I almost immediately began to feel better. It was as if someone had flipped a switch on my health meter. I wondered, Why did I start feeling so sick just before Christmas, and now that it was over, I quickly felt so much better? What was it about Christmas? Was it the cold? The snow? The stress?

As I thought about it more, I recognized that this same thing had happened to me last year at about the same time. It wasn't as dramatic, but I hadn't felt well last year at Christmastime, either. I'd had the same flu-like symptoms—headaches, muscle pain, earaches, and brain fog—and, yes, the symptoms had quickly subsided after Christmas. What could cause this to happen both years at the same time?

Could it be . . . the Christmas tree?

From the moment the idea popped into my head, it made so much sense. My allergies to hay and ragweed were so intense, so wouldn't it make sense that I could be allergic to pine trees, too? I'd never heard of such a thing, though, so could this really be true?

As soon as I told Mary about the possibility, she began to do some research. Allergies to Christmas trees were actually quite common, she discovered. Some people even died from an allergic response to their tree! People could be allergic to the pine tree itself or to the mold that often came into the house along with the tree. It amazed both of us that something so common could be so dangerous, yet neither of us had ever heard any warnings about it. It was obvious that we had to get rid of the tree, so we did.

As my brain continued to clear and my body returned to better health, I continued to contemplate my situation. If I was allergic to the tree—or its mold—why was my response this year so strong compared to how I'd felt in years past? Perhaps my immune system was stronger then, or maybe the effect upon our household was simply less dramatic because Mary was less stressed at that time and thus better able to cope with the bulk of the responsibilities. I'll probably never know, but one thing was clear: we'd never have a live Christmas tree in our home again.

As the new year progressed, the symptoms I'd felt in response to the Christmas tree lessened. Nonetheless, I began to notice increased pressure in my head that was different from the headache I'd felt before. Taking a cue from what I'd learned from the Christmas tree—the notion that everything I put in me and everything around me might cause me to feel ill—I began to wonder if the drops prescribed by the allergist in LaCrosse might be the cause. So I stopped taking them and almost immediately experienced relief. After a few days, I took the drops, and the tension in my head returned. *Great*, I thought. *I am allergic to my allergy medication. What are the odds?*

When I called the allergist and explained the situation, the doctor confirmed that the right thing to do was to stop taking the sublingual drops I'd been prescribed. Unfortunately, he also explained that since I was reacting to them, there wasn't anything else he could do to help me. So although I was relieved to find the cause of this latest discomfort, it was clear that I'd come to the end of another road that I'd once hoped could fully restore my health. I knew I still needed to find someone who could do that, but I didn't have any idea about where to turn. Once again, I was forced to take a deep breath and hope that something would one day be revealed.

The ups and downs of my health in this new year mimicked the relationship between Mary and me at the same time. There were some good moments and some bad ones. Still, just beneath the surface, there was almost always a level of tension that led to frequent arguments—or silence—between us. One didn't have to look too deep to see we were just getting by, yet both of us were almost too tired to care. I needed Mary to comfort me; she needed me to help her. We were both too drained, however, to give the other what was needed.

At that time, my job involved standing and occasionally walking on hard concrete floors for nearly eight hours long, five days a week. Other than the two twenty-minute breaks I was allotted, there were no opportunities to sit down. So by the end of the day, my legs were in a great deal of pain. I suppose that's the case for many who work in similar conditions, but from what I could surmise, the pain I felt was beyond that of most others. Once I got home and was finally able to sit, it was both mentally and physically difficult for me to get up.

Mary was exhausted, too, albeit for different reasons and in different ways. Her job as a teacher was emotionally challenging and involved a lengthy list of responsibilities. She typically worked ten-hour days and went back to school on the weekends to do even more. I knew she needed my help with responsibilities at home, so I tried to take care of the kids, tidy up, and make the evening meal during the week. By sitting on a chair or even the floor wherever I could, I was usually able to muster the strength to do what was needed. Still, it was tough. Really tough.

One day, Mary came home a little earlier than I'd expected. When she saw me sitting on the floor by the stove, drying some dishes while cooking dinner, she flipped out. In her eyes, I was once again over-dramatizing my situation, making a show of things to garner sympathy or just to be lazy. It didn't help that outside of the allergist in LaCrosse, none of the many doctors I'd seen had been able to confirm my symptoms or diagnose any type of illness. So I'm sure there was at least some doubt in Mary's own head about whether or not I was as incapacitated as I acted. Mary would surely have been more understanding and comforting if she weren't as tired and frustrated herself, but that wasn't her reality at the time. We were obviously both doing the best we could.

It was at about this time that I stopped taking the Sulfasalazine I'd been taking for the ulcerative colitis I'd been diagnosed with several years earlier. I don't quite know how it came about. Maybe my prescription ran out, and I just put off getting it refilled. Or maybe, like with the Christmas tree and the allergy drops, I began to wonder about its effect on me and decided to put it to the test. Sure enough, after several days, the brutal discomfort in my legs began to subside. After a few weeks, I couldn't believe the difference. I was thrilled—but also worried. My legs now felt better, but without the medicine, how was I going to prevent painful flare-ups from occurring?

When I contacted the doctor to tell him about my situation, I was hopeful there would be another medication I could substitute for the Sulfasalazine. Unfortunately, since I hadn't been seen by her in quite some time and since I hadn't followed through with her recommendation for bi-yearly colonoscopies to help her monitor the situation, she insisted upon this procedure before she would even see me. Of course, there was no alternative but to do just what she asked. So I scheduled the procedure and got it over with as soon as possible. When I met with her shortly afterward, she surprised me by telling me how healthy my colon appeared and that while there was some sign of the disease, it was very moderate. She then prescribed a new medication and sent me on my way.

Within a week of starting the new medication, a familiar discomfort began to appear in my legs and even in my lower back. When it continued to worsen, I once again decided to stop taking the medication. At that time, in fact, I chose to stop taking medication for the ulcerative colitis altogether—if only just to give myself a break from the discomfort and time to figure out if there were any other options for me. Of course, without any medication, I'd have to be especially careful about what I ate in order to keep from irritating my colon. I wasn't sure how I was going to do that since I had already limited my diet quite a bit. Moreover, I wasn't even sure that the foods I thought were safe actually would be without any medication at all.

My legs were better, but I was mentally and emotionally exhausted. I knew I wasn't pleasant to be around most of the time and required more care and patience than Mary had to give. We were nearing a breaking point, both individually and as a couple, but we didn't know where or how to find some relief. Many times, it seemed like it would have been easier just to give up.

Chapter 10

Swimming Upstream

*The afflictions of the righteous are many,
but the Lord rescues him from them all.*
Psalm 34:19

In addition to the stress brought about by my illness, our family was further impacted by the financial damage that came with it. Frequent trips to the doctor, along with various attempts with supplements and other uninsured treatments suggested by friends, seen on social media, or noticed through the research Mary was doing for me, seriously affected our bank account on what seemed like a regular basis. We were desperate for something positive to occur. Still, day after day, the same routine struggles came and went. Until one day, that is, when a bit of good news did arrive in the form of a unique Christmas gift: an invitation to join Mary's family for a week-long vacation in Myrtle Beach, South Carolina, with all expenses to be paid by her parents. It appeared to be just what we needed.

The trip would occur in late March, which was the time that most Wisconsinites have had just about enough of the snow and chill that seem to linger far too long into spring. Mary had visions of relaxing on a sunny beach while I couldn't help but look forward to a few rounds of golf. We both were excited for an opportunity to relieve ourselves from the daily grind.

After several months of anticipation, the day of our flight finally arrived. We felt well-prepared for the trip as we buckled everyone into the car in the early morning hours and waved goodbye to our home as we headed off on the ninety-mile drive to the airport. We'd been on the road for less than thirty minutes when Joe, who was eighteen months old at the time, threw up in the car. He must have had a big breakfast because it was all over him, his car seat, and the surrounding area. We shrugged off the stress and tried to make light of the situation as Mary changed his clothes while I wiped up his seat and the surrounding area as well as possible. He wasn't acting sick and didn't appear to have a fever, so we crossed our fingers that the incident was just a fluke and continued on our way.

We continued to watch Joe carefully during the remainder of the trip. Thankfully, he appeared to be just fine . . . until we pulled into the airport's parking garage, where Joe suddenly began Round Two. From the sound, it appeared to be even worse than the first time. We pulled into a spot as quickly as possible and jumped out of the car to assess things more carefully. Flicking on the overhead light, I saw the nasty evidence that confirmed my initial response. Instinctively, Mary took Joe and began to change his clothes. Meanwhile, I gathered the seat cover, blanket, and miscellaneous items I'd used to wipe up around the area and put them all in a bag in our luggage to be dealt with later.

At this point, we began to seriously question what to do. Should we turn around and go back home or change it and continue with our original plans? Joe was once again sound asleep and still without any sign of a fever. We were still on time for our flight, and we still had visions of sun, warmth, and opportunity ahead. Furthermore, the thought of wasting several hundred dollars' worth of airline tickets to return home, where Joe may not actually have any additional signs of illness, seemed quite possible. A decision had to be made, and since we couldn't see into the future to know whether it was a good one or a bad one, we decided to stay the course and continue our journey.

The boarding process occurred without a hitch, and we were soon buckling ourselves into our seats on the plane and preparing for takeoff. Joe rested quietly in Mary's arms while I helped Julia get situated in her seat. The excitement of watching Julia experience her first airplane flight was almost enough to distract us from our challenging morning. We were also comforted by the thought that regardless of what happened from this point on, it wouldn't be long before we would arrive in Myrtle Beach where Joe could get some quality rest, then (hopefully) wake up refreshed and ready to go to the beach.

A layover in Cincinnati involved a short wait before boarding the plane to our final destination. We'd originally planned to have time to get some breakfast before our first flight but had scrapped that plan due to the unexpected circumstances we'd encountered. So by now, we were rather hungry. Lucky for us, we found ourselves waiting for our next flight right beside a pizza kiosk, and it smelled delicious. I knew that my stomach couldn't tolerate any, but I was sure that Mary and Julia would appreciate a slice or two.

Everyone else must have been thinking the same thing because the line for the pizza stretched way out into the walkway. I calculated that there was likely just enough time for me to get them each a slice, so I made sure they were comfortable and headed over to join the line. It wasn't fast, but the prize seemed well worth the wait. I moved along with it slowly and made it to the counter just as boarding began for the first seats on our flight. "Two slices of pepperoni!" I announced to the teenager behind the counter while keeping my eyes on the flight attendant who was announcing which passengers were now eligible to be seated. "Oh, I'm sorry, sir," he said. "We just ran out of pizza. All we have left are beverages. What can I get you to drink?" "Are you SERIOUS?" I groaned. The clerk just looked at me expressionless and nodded. I wanted to climb over the counter and take a look myself—there had to be *something* back there to eat. I didn't want anything to drink. I wanted something to *eat,* even if it wasn't for me. Even if I got some pizza, I still wouldn't even have anything for ME. All I could do was turn away and walk dejectedly back to my family . . . with no pizza.

Trying to cheer everyone up, I said at least there would be peanuts on the plane and reminded them that we had the warmth and sunshine of South Carolina ahead of us. As we settled into our seats for the next flight, I saw that Joe was resting comfortably in Mary's arms. I took a moment to consider how thankful I was that our rough start seemed to have evened out a bit. Once we were in the air, Julia and I looked out the window and talked about the patchwork of fields below, dissected by roads and interspersed with waterways, towns, and cities. The awe and wonder of flight at such a young age were reflected in her eyes.

When our plane neared the airport, the pilot's voice came over the intercom, and we assumed we were about to hear the typical end-of-flight announcements. Unfortunately, this wasn't the case. Instead, the pilot coolly announced that it was too foggy to land the plane at this time, so we'd be circling the airfield for a while until the weather cleared. The kids were quiet and didn't seem to mind, so it was easy for us to be okay with the change. An hour later, the pilot spoke to us once again, but the news this time was unsettling. Apparently, it was still too foggy for a safe landing in Myrtle Beach, so the flight was being diverted to an airport in Columbia, South Carolina, instead. A bus would meet us there to bring us back to our original destination. Although disappointed and still hungry, I reminded myself to be grateful that Joe was still sleeping comfortably and had no fever. At least we could now say we'd been to Columbia!

When we landed in Columbia, I jumped up quickly to grab our things and take Julia's hand. We headed to pick up our bags, then hustled to the bus pick-up area. We sure didn't want to miss that! When we arrived outside, where we were told the bus would be waiting, our eyes scanned the lot but saw nothing and no one. There was no sign that we were in the right place and no one to ask. Eventually, though, a few other groups of people meandered to the area and confirmed for us that they'd been on the flight too and were also waiting for transportation to Myrtle Beach. There was soon a small crowd gathered around us, all waiting for the bus, but no bus came. Some kids nearby pulled out a deck of Uno cards while others colored in a coloring book, and the adults waited quietly. Finally, two hours later, one of the group members called out, "There it is!" Sure enough, a bus was headed our way. Was it ours, though?

Thankfully, the bus came near and eventually stopped right in front of us. When the door opened, we poked our heads inside and asked the driver if he was sent to take us to Myrtle Beach. He nodded his head and made his way down the steps to open the large luggage doors on the side of the bus. Mary and I scooped up our belongings and bolted to the curb, hoping we could instigate haste from the rest of the crowd by being speedy ourselves. The driver took our bags, tossed them in the bin, and then turned his attention to the rest of the group as we hustled toward the bus door. We climbed up the steps and plopped ourselves expectantly into the first row of seats. As we almost simultaneously let out a deep sigh of relief, we noticed a beautiful sunset developing beyond the large windshield in front of us. It was as if God had painted an amazing picture to sustain our tired, hungry, and otherwise frustrated little family. It was just what we needed. We smiled at each other, snuggled Julia between us, and settled Joe into a position that would help him continue to sleep comfortably throughout this next step of our journey.

It was dark and surprisingly chilly when we arrived in Myrtle Beach almost four hours later. Since cell phones weren't yet available, we weren't sure what the rest of Mary's family knew about the status of our flight and bus trip and how they'd reacted to it. They'd flown there a few days earlier and had originally planned to meet us at the airport with a rented car to bring us to the condo, but with the change, we weren't sure if that was still the case. Almost as soon as we exited the bus, however, we heard Mary's parents call our names and saw them waiting nearby. They were all smiles as we approached, and they chuckled as we discussed the day's events. It was hard to return their enthusiasm and good cheer, however, because we were tired, frustrated, and still a little worried about Joe. Nevertheless, we tried to match their excited chatter as we moved through the city and eventually arrived at the condo. When we pulled into the driveway, we noticed my brother-in-law removing the last pieces of luggage from the trunk of his car. He'd beaten us here even though he'd chosen to drive rather than fly, and we'd left our homes at nearly the same time that same morning. It was pretty annoying, to be honest.

Once we had settled in, we warmed. Then we ate the leftover supper that had been made several hours earlier, talked a little with the family, then headed off to bed. Joe was still lethargic but didn't have a temperature and hadn't vomited since early in the day, so we were hopeful that he was on the mend. I was planning to join much of the family for a round of golf early the next morning, and Mary was planning to sleep in and enjoy time with the kids at the condo and on the beach.

One of the first things I did when I woke up the next morning was to check in with Joe. He'd slept through the night and was still without a fever but had a pretty good case of diarrhea. It looked like he'd need another day or so to return to good health, so the beach would likely have to wait. Hopefully, though, the worst was behind us. I gave Mary a few words of encouragement and a quick hug, then grabbed my cap and headed out the door.

When I returned from the golf course several hours later, Julia was on the balcony blowing bubbles in the wind, my in-laws were making small talk around the table, and Mary was sitting stone-faced on the couch holding Joe. Although it wasn't yet noon, I could tell she was already at the end of her rope. I tried to lighten her mood, but my attempts returned only cold eyes and sharp words. What she didn't verbalize then, she unleashed later in private. She was tired, worried about Joe, and upset that she had been left alone with him while I was out playing golf. Moreover, she was frustrated by the weather, which (despite what we'd planned) was irritatingly rainy and cold, and was hardly able to contain the toxic feelings of sibling rivalry she so often felt when she was with her brother and sisters. She clearly needed a break. I took Joe from her and tried to find appropriate, comforting words, but it was clear that there wasn't much I could do.

I wish I could say that our faith in God and each other prevailed and that all of our troubles melted away in light of our spiritual conviction, but we had so much more growing to do. God was sharpening us to serve Him and each other more fully, but being sharpened is difficult and not much fun. While we were unquestionably blessed by much during our "vacation," we didn't do a good job of appreciating it because we let ourselves be frustrated by things we felt hadn't aligned with what we'd wanted or expected. All we noticed was the negative: how Joe remained sick for almost the entire week; how the wind howled and the sun didn't shine until the very last day we were there; how we had to wait several hours at the airport before our flight home because it was delayed by high winds; how, when we'd finally arrived back in Wisconsin, the car battery was dead because I'd forgotten to switch off the interior light after turning it on to clean up Joe's mess; and how the serviceman's portable car jump starter was broken when he arrived, and it took him two hours to find another one. The point is that in not trusting God, we saw only the negative side of almost everything we experienced during our trip, which caused us to sacrifice the joy and peace that certainly were available to us, albeit somewhat hard to find. Today I'm better at seeking the positive in negative situations, and while it's something I have to make a conscious choice to do, it's still not easy!

Chapter 11

Contagious Pessimism

The Lord is my shepherd, I will not be in need. He lets me lie down in green pastures; He leads me beside quiet waters. He restores my soul; he guides me in the paths of righteousness for the sake of His name. Even though I walk through the valley of the shadow of death, I fear no evil, for You are with me; Your rod and Your staff, they comfort me.
Psalm 23:1-4

Getting away to Myrtle Beach had been a change of scenery and routine, even though it was one of those vacations where one doesn't really rest. Upon our return, we fell back into our usual routine pretty quickly, but with a little better dynamic between Mary and me—for the moment, at least. Eventually, I found myself slipping into a new negative thought pattern, *Why can't anything just go right for once?*

One night, shortly after our trip, I experienced something I still don't understand. I was just dozing off when I heard an extremely loud BANG! I sprang up in bed and, wide-eyed, looked around the room. Mary was still asleep next to me. The house was dark and still. There wasn't anything out of place. As I looked and listened, nothing was taking place to cause concern. After a few seconds, I concluded the sound was just in my head. *But what could possibly have triggered such a sudden and loud noise?*

It took me a while to get back to sleep that night. Between worrying about what had occurred and waiting for it to happen again, I didn't get much rest. When I discussed it with Mary the next morning, our conversation led me to wonder if the noise I'd heard had only been in my head. Could it be yet another strange health issue? Mary did a quick internet search and, to our surprise, quickly uncovered a condition aptly named Exploding Head Syndrome (EHS). Apparently, EHS is a very rare sensory disorder whose exact cause is unknown. It is hypothesized to be the result of miscommunication between neurons in the brain due to anxiety, stress, minor seizures in the temporal lobe, middle ear issues, or because of reactions to medications, among other things. I sighed, wrestling with the confirmation of yet one more crazy medical symptom.

The next night, it was hard for me to relax because I was anxious that I'd have another instance of EHS. Thankfully, I eventually fell asleep and enjoyed a peaceful rest that night and for many nights afterward. When a couple of weeks passed, it seemed I was in the clear, and I forgot about it. Then it happened again, and my cycle of worry began again. During that period of time, I had about a dozen episodes of EHS, but for some reason I haven't had any more, even to this day. That's a strange reality I've experienced many times in my life: I have a strange and uncomfortable physical sensation that occurs for a while (sometimes a long while and sometimes for just a brief period of time), then goes away. Sometimes it comes back, and other times it doesn't. Like so much else, it seems inexplicable.

I know it's devastating for millions of people in the world who visit the doctor and receive a critical, negative diagnosis about their condition, but although I've expected that many, many times, it was never the case for me. My routine was to feel ill, see the doctor, and then be sent home after being told that I was perfectly healthy, which over time became traumatic for me in its own way. As if to top things off, it was occasionally implied that although my physical health was perfect, my mental state was likely less so. I knew that what I was feeling was *not* just "in my head." Hence, I began to assume that this was the standard response when a physician simply didn't know what else to say; when the tests didn't show abnormal levels to indicate a specific condition, or the symptoms I mentioned didn't ring a bell in their minds about a particular disorder. It would have been easier to believe if one or more of the physicians had at least asked for a moment to refer to a medical journal or requested a few days so they could do some research about my condition, but that *never* occurred—not once by a general practitioner and not once by a specialist. It was almost as if I and the other patients in a clinic were simply place keepers on a mechanical belt being run past the doctors in a clinic. The patient was plopped in a room, questioned by a nurse, then visited by the physician, who then proclaimed a diagnosis and sent the patient out the door so this could be repeated with the next individual—all within a fifteen-minute period of time. Were we all just cogs in the system? Shouldn't medical treatment be more than this?

Ironically, the fact that I felt ignored and unimportant by so many physicians led me to develop emotional issues that otherwise may not have occurred. It's difficult to put into words how hard it is to cope when you're feeling miserable and seem to have nowhere to turn to find relief. It appeared that there wasn't even one physician who wanted to hear about my problems. What's more, after a while, my friends didn't want to hear about them, my siblings didn't want to hear about them, and even Mary was worn out from hearing about them. I couldn't have felt more alone.

Since I looked healthy on the outside, those around me expected me to act that way. I tried—I really did. I started taking Sulfasalazine again (which I'd previously stopped because it made my legs feel so tired and in hopes that I could then expand my food choices). Every day, I got up and went to work just like everybody else I knew. During these years, in addition to what I was expected to accomplish at work each day, I had to struggle every minute just to stay upright and alert. Looking back, I often wonder how I did it. It could only have been the grace of God.

With new issues constantly appearing, an underlying despair began to creep into my heart. What was to become of me? Would all of these symptoms continue to pile on until I was absolutely buried in them? What would that look like? What would that feel like? How would I be able to cope with all of this as I aged when even the healthiest body loses its vigor? It was obvious no one could really understand what was going on with me, and even if they did—what could they really do to help me? My present discomfort and worry about the future caused me to become even more short-tempered with my co-workers, more easily frustrated with Mary, and certainly not a whole lot of fun for my kids to be around.

Problems between Mary and I began to escalate. When I forced myself to get out and do things with her, I usually regretted it even before we'd arrived at our destination. I could focus only on how long it would be before we could return home. Whenever I could, wherever we were, I sought opportunities to find a quiet place to lie down and relax. I rarely smiled, cried often and frequently, and as soon as we were out of earshot of others (and sometimes not waiting until then), scolded Mary about why she'd talked to an acquaintance after church, why she'd spent so long saying goodbye to her family, or why she'd left me alone for so much of the time. This, of course, only drove a wedge deeper between Mary and me.

It wasn't too difficult to notice how my physical condition had changed me. I was once a guy who loved socializing and sought out an adventure. Now, however, I just wanted to go home and to bed where it was quiet. I wasn't the least bit interested in doing anything beyond my usual daily routine, and I usually didn't feel like sharing my time or effort unless there was something in it for me. Most of all, I was utterly and completely without hope.

As you might imagine, life for Mary at this point wasn't easy or happy either. It would have been understandable for her to leave me like my mom had left my dad, but she was devoted to our family and honored the bond with which God had joined us. Since there was so much in her life that she couldn't control because of my health issues, she'd learned to live without asking for much in return. There was something she did want, however: another baby.

With all of my physical difficulties, I wasn't interested in complicating things any further by adding another child to our family. Still, Mary was persistent. She talked about it all the time, and I mostly listened but gave my point of view frequently enough that she knew where I stood on the matter. Naturally, my opinion made her unhappy, and that made me unhappy. Then, in July of 1999, Mary approached me with a sly smile and told me she was pregnant. I later discovered that she believed I'd be happy if it happened, even though I'd indicated otherwise beforehand. It turns out she was right. I had no idea how we would cope, not only financially but with the added responsibility. Nonetheless, there was no doubt that I was excited. Obviously, Mary was happy, too, and that made life easier for me.

Stephen was born in February of 2000. In spite of my stress, physical afflictions, and general exhaustion, I was instantly filled with joy. Stephen was beautiful! I didn't celebrate by going golfing with my buddies the next day like I'd done with my other children. Though to be completely honest, it was February, and the weather wasn't conducive to playing golf. If it had been summertime, though, I like to think that I'd learned something from my previous experiences and wanted to make better choices this time. So I stayed with Mary at the hospital, helped her with Julia and Joe as much as possible upon our arrival home, and ground my way through fatigue and pain to help prepare meals and tidy the house throughout the following weeks. I still didn't get up in the middle of the night to change a diaper or bring the baby to Mary for a feeding. By then, though, Mary had given up on trying to get me to help in that way, so she didn't even ask.

When Stephen was born, Julia was five, and Joe was three and a half. All of our children have brought us joy, each in their own unique way. Julia was a beautiful baby and cute toddler who was almost always gentle and considerate. Joe was a little charmer who was cute and cuddly, and I recall early on how smart he was—and how stubborn! Stephen was the perfect third child. He didn't cry a lot and didn't need a lot to stay happy. For a guy like me with so many other problems, Stephen was a definite Godsend.

Of course, while Stephen's arrival was a blessing, it couldn't change my miserable health. However, it was at this time that my discomfort led to a realization: just when I felt like I could take no more of one health issue or another, it would fade away, and something else would take its place. This seemed to occur on a seasonal basis. For example, in August, ragweed pollen overwhelmed my body and led to all kinds of issues. I would feel progressively worse until it seemed like I couldn't take it anymore. Then the weather would turn colder, which would eliminate the pollen and lighten the load on my body until mid-winter.

Unfortunately, because the house was now closed up tightly, I was greatly affected by dust mites, which brought continual flu-like symptoms and a complete lack of energy. When the weather became warm again, I spent more time outside, where the fresh air and sunshine began to revive me. Mid-summer was always the best time of the year. My neck was not as stiff, my head didn't ache as much, and I had more energy. I could also tolerate a greater variety of foods. Needless to say, I was always healthiest—and happiest—in July.

Not every day was a July day, and when it wasn't, life was more challenging and unpleasant than I wanted to bear. By default, Mary often viewed life in the same way. We grappled with the weight of caring for three young children, managing the responsibility of home ownership, holding down two full-time jobs, and constantly dealing with my compromised health, which regularly depleted our money and energy. My depleted health wasn't just a burden on me; it was extremely troublesome to Mary, too. Where she needed a husband's comfort, understanding, and support, she had me, who didn't have any to give.

Although Mary had once told me that she'd known right away that I was the one for her, things had clearly changed. She no longer looked at me the way she used to, and she didn't respond to me like she had before. Where my wife had once admired my strength and independence, she had come to see me as weak and needy. I couldn't blame her. I felt that way about myself.

On the one hand, I couldn't blame Mary for the fact that her love for me had eroded, but on the other, it made me spiteful and desperate. My anger about the situation increased the frequency and intensity of our arguments. Mary began to say things I never expected to hear, and I quickly responded with equal cruelty. We did our best to forgive and forget between the fights, but the arguments troubled both of us. The probability of a successful outcome for this marriage frightened both of us.

Chapter 12

An Unexpected Gift

For this reason I too, having heard of the faith in the Lord Jesus which exists among you and [a] your love for all the saints, do not cease giving thanks for you, while making mention of you in my prayers; that the God of our Lord Jesus Christ, the Father of glory, may give you a spirit of wisdom and of revelation in the knowledge of Him.
Ephesians 1:15-17

I hadn't realized how much I'd needed Mary up to that point; I was too preoccupied with being worn down and feeling sorry for myself. I'd been overdrawing our relationship account for years. They say God doesn't bring you to a place without helping you through it, and I don't think I fully appreciated how He'd done that with Mary in my life.

One day while shopping in a store that sold educational materials for teachers, she noticed a sign advertising counseling services for children and adults with learning disabilities. For years she had maintained there was more to my learning difficulties than simple stupidity. When she saw this sign, she began to push me to have the problem diagnosed. She believed, if nothing else, that evaluation by a professional and the appropriate support would enable me to better manage the challenge.

I wasn't as hopeful as Mary. In fact, the whole thing dredged up feelings of anger, injustice, and resentment. Whereas I'd have given just about anything to uncover what was wrong with me physically, I wasn't as keen to know what had made learning so difficult for me in school. *Someone should have taken the time to find this out long ago.* I frowned. *Somebody should have made the effort to help me before I had to endure years of frustration and humiliation in front of my peers. Maybe then my self-esteem would have remained intact, and my life would have turned out to be less disappointing.* Nevertheless, I realized there was another reason I didn't want to know more about this: maybe it would reveal that I was just plain dumb. I'd always felt that way growing up, and I certainly didn't need to load that pile of disappointment onto my shoulders at this point in my life.

Mary's educator instincts, though, demanded some deeper answers. She encouraged me by telling me that if I were diagnosed with a learning disability, I could unlock the door to specific actions that could possibly help me. I couldn't really argue with that. *At the very least, I want to give her hope for some kind of improvement in this life of ours,* I reasoned. So after dragging my feet for a few weeks, I reluctantly agreed to set up an appointment.

The counselor was a big man but was soft-spoken and had a gentle attitude. After some small talk, he asked me to read a few paragraphs aloud. While I did so, he listened intently and scribbled some notes. He then asked me a few questions about what I'd read and had me do some writing. When I was done, he took a look at my work, then put his notepad and my writing aside. He then looked up at me, smiled, and began to speak.

"John," he said, "you have a disorder that makes it difficult for you to read or interpret letters, words, and other symbols." He explained that I wasn't dumb, but that reading and writing were just more difficult for me than it was for most other people. He told me there were lots of people who had this same condition and that there was an official name for the disorder: dyslexia.

As exciting as it was to know that there was a valid reason for my learning challenges that were beyond my control, it was also extremely irritating. Of all the people in the world that could have had it, why did it have to be *me*? Moreover, if I had to be one of the unlucky ones with dyslexia, why didn't anyone know about it for my entire school career? Why did I have to endure years of humiliation in school when that time was supposed to have been used to make my life better? It wasn't fair.

For the problem solver Mary, however, this news was a spark of opportunity. She was instantly emboldened to help me find a way to use the diagnosis to my advantage. After a little research, we learned that the United States provides legal protection for people diagnosed with dyslexia and that financial support is available for further education if it is something that hinders one at work. Mary also encouraged me to use the word to describe myself to others as a way of advocating for myself when it was needed. Instead of trying to hide the fact I struggled to read and write, I just explained to others I was dyslexic and moved on. It was strangely freeing.

After a few sessions with the counselor, Mary found a few more resources she thought might be helpful. One of them was an opportunity for reading instruction through The Davis Dyslexia Program. There were several practitioners around the country trained in this protocol. The nearest one, however, was based in Milwaukee, which was a ninety-minute drive from us. The program was also fairly expensive. Thankfully, though, Mary discovered that my employer funded employee education. I also discovered that I'd earned an additional week of vacation that year due to my longevity with the company, so it seemed like the perfect opportunity to jump in. For my part, spending what should have been a week of vacation solely on reading and writing didn't sound like a vacation at all. Still, it did appear to be a beneficial opportunity—and Mary was so excited about it that I didn't want to disappoint her.

In truth, there were a few other reasons why I felt that this might not be so bad. For one, I'd get a break from eight hours of standing on the cement floors at the plant. In addition, I'd get to enjoy ninety minutes listening to some good old seventies and eighties classics during the drive. The main reason I agreed to the program, though, was because I didn't want to let Mary down. After all, without a good excuse, it would have appeared that I wasn't interested in trying to improve myself. So even though I was the one going, and even though I wasn't sure I was the one *needing* me to go, I went anyway.

Besides improving my ability to read and write, hearing the theory about *why* I'd struggled to do so was the deeper reward. My tutor began by identifying two key components of my condition. Component number one was my focus—or lack of it. A big part of the problem was my racing mind. She explained my brain moves through two or more times as many images per second than a "regular" brain does. Also, although "regular" brains occasionally pause, brains like mine just go and go and go, bouncing from one thought to another, never stopping.

The second component of my condition was the richness with which I visualized things. My tutor explained that when I read, write, or hear about something, I automatically create three-dimensional images of it. Most people with "regular" brains visualize images that are only two-dimensional. Furthermore, since my mind is continually in motion (component number one), it takes the three-dimensional image and views it from all angles, moves it from one place to another, and even utilizes it for different purposes. As you can imagine, it can be pretty difficult for me to focus on reading or writing when all of this hyperactivity is going on in my head.

I think I'd always known I had a fast-moving brain and saw things as three-dimensional images that I was constantly manipulating, so that wasn't really a revelation to me. What *was* intriguing was that this was *not* how other people's brains worked. Imagine my surprise when my tutor explained that the mind of a dyslexic was actually *a gift*. She told me that dyslexics are often the first ones to demonstrate out-of-the-box thinking; they are inventors and problem solvers who do work that is difficult and often not even possible for those with "regular" brains. I could actually relate to this a bit because I knew that I'd been able to excel at work by identifying solutions that others couldn't see. I wasn't aware, however, that this was actually a gift. I'd *never* considered the workings of my brain to be a gift. After all, even if my brain was as wonderful as she said it was, if a person couldn't read or write because of its uniqueness, it was hard to view it as anything other than a hindrance to success.

My tutor clarified how a dyslexic's mind works by explaining that an individual with dyslexia would likely not have trouble reading and understanding a sentence like "My dog ran." This is because each word in the sentence can be visualized. "My" is me, which I can visualize. I can also create an image for a "dog," and I can certainly see that the dog "ran." Not a problem. She continued, however, stating that it can be difficult for a dyslexic to read and understand a sentence like "I see a dog running over to that car." Mental images can be created for each of the words at the beginning of the sentence, "I see a dog running." When the reader gets to the words "to" and "that," however, there isn't an image to be created. This is where the reader begins to struggle—not so much because he or she can't read the words, but because there aren't visual representations for them. Compounding the problem is component number one again: the fact that a dyslexic's mind never stops. So when one of those non-visual words is met, and no meaning is matched with them, the mind doesn't stop to re-evaluate. Instead, it moves on to something else, which is likely not related to the original words on the page. It was easy to see how this quickly became a problem.

I wondered what magic cure the Davis Dyslexia Program would use to help people like me. According to my teacher, the answer was to give a visual meaning to those seemingly meaningless connecting words—words like "the," "of," and "but." She began training me to memorize the "official" definition for each of those words from the dictionary. Once the definition was memorized, I worked a piece of clay into an object that represented that specific word to me. The memorization of the definition, along with the clay representation, gave visual meaning to the word. This meant that when I came to that word in my reading, my mind was now able to picture it and comprehend it. Thus, I was able to maintain my focus and my comprehension of the sentence. Hallelujah! It sounded almost too good to be true.

During our time together, my tutor and I found time to discuss other things too. We talked about our families, which eventually led to me sharing about my physical ailments and my frustration about not being able to find any answers. At some point, I mentioned that I loved God but had a lot of questions for Him, such as why He would allow me to suffer for so long like I did. She responded with words of empathy and shared that she was also a Christian. She'd read and studied the Bible many times and began to share with me how she interpreted His message for us through The Good Book. We had many conversations that week during the down times before, during, and after the lessons, which inspired me and awakened a curiosity in me about the Bible that I hadn't previously recognized. On my last day, she presented me with a complete audio set of the Bible that she'd purchased for me at a local bookstore during her lunch break. Her generosity surprised me, and although I appreciated it, I wasn't yet aware of how valuable that gift would become to me.

After completing the in-class portion of the program, I was sent home with tasks similar to those I'd done with my tutor that would help me continue to improve my reading ability. The thought, however, of having to practice and memorize each and every word that didn't have an innate meaning behind it felt more than a little daunting, not just because of the volume of words that I would need to master but also because of the demands of my young family and constantly challenged health.

The week-long program had exhausted me, so I took the weekend and the following week off to rest but planned to begin working again soon after. When the time came, though, my health once again began to spiral downward. I put aside my homework and tried to simply garner the strength and endurance to make it through each day. During this period, more than one co-worker, friend, and family member remarked to me that I didn't look well. Some even went so far as to tell me that I looked like I was dying. I couldn't disagree. My skin had a pale, almost grayish pallor; I was losing weight and had very low energy. Whether I looked like it or not, I sure felt like I was dying—and it was a slow and painful death.

At this point, perhaps more than ever before, nearly everything around me seemed to have an adverse effect on my body. By now, I'd learned to be very careful about what I ate, drank, and put on my body. Still, apparently avoiding any one previously-identified culprit wasn't enough. Some things didn't seem to affect me one day but bothered me another, so I began to consider other possibilities. Perhaps my body wasn't affected by a one-time exposure to an item but only noticeably troubled after a second, third, or fourth encounter with it. Or perhaps it wasn't any one item alone but instead the combination of two or more items. Or maybe my body reacted when an item was prepared with a different preservative or prepared somewhat differently than in another instance. Maybe my body was reacting to pesticide infiltration of a product or genetic modification of some of its ingredients. Maybe my body was more easily overwhelmed one day compared to another because of other allergens that were stressing me at that time, such as mold in the soil of the house plants, dust mites in the carpet, mercury in my fillings, and/or plastic fumes in the plant where I worked. Or maybe my body was affected by environmental allergens, a lack of sunshine, or negative or positive ions in the air. Was my body bothered by the supplements I was taking or affected because of a lack of a different kind of element? Was it a little or a lot of some random variation of these factors? Or was it none of these things?

Unfortunately, no one seemed to know, and there didn't seem to be anyone else to ask. I needed to do something—but what? The first thing I did was try to pare down my life to its most basic form. I thought that by simplifying my life, I could perhaps notice what negatively affected me. So once again, I stopped taking all the Sulfasalazine along with the supplements I'd been taking, drank only filtered water, purchased hypoallergenic products whenever possible, and trimmed my diet to the barest of essentials. Mary purchased additional dust-mite-resistant coverings, got rid of every houseplant in our home, and bought an air purifier for our bedroom.

The most immediate result seemed to come from the suspension of the medication I was taking for the ulcerative colitis. In only a few days, I began to look and feel a lot better. Of course, I still felt pretty sick—like I had just one foot in the grave instead of two—but at least people stopped telling me I looked like I was dying.

When I contacted the doctor that had prescribed the medicine, I was basically told that it was inexcusable to forgo taking medication for ulcerative colitis once it had been diagnosed. Since Mary and I had recently read about how the health of one's stomach can affect the overall health of one's body, it seemed plausible that the doctor's point of view was accurate; medication was essential. My physician assured me that even if I chose not to take the originally-prescribed medicine, there were other medicines that could be substituted for it. So he prescribed another and then another as I bounced from prescription to prescription, trying to find one that wouldn't affect me so negatively. Unfortunately, all of them seemed to be as bad as the first—not right away, but after a few days or weeks of time. Despite what the doctor said, my health seemed better without the medication than with it.

Once I realized how much better I felt without the medication, which the doctor had assured me was not in my best interest, I began to reconsider whether or not the doctor really had my best interest in mind. Like most Americans, I'd been raised to believe that if there was a medical problem, it could be resolved—or at least identified—by a doctor. Even so, my faith in the system had definitely started to dim. Perhaps, though, this was just because the doctors in my small town didn't have enough experience or knowledge to address the really difficult cases. Maybe a doctor in a bigger city or more prestigious clinic would be able to help me. Actually, looking elsewhere was my only choice at this point because I'd been to all the local physicians, and they'd not only been unable to help me but had typically sent me away, sure that my problems were related to my mental health rather than anything physical.

Mary began to schedule appointments for me out of town with new doctors that were highly regarded—at least according to the reviews on the internet. Each time, I sent my records ahead with the hope that the physician I'd be seeing would study my situation and be prepared to offer me relevant advice. Unfortunately, that was never the case. It seemed that each time the doctor walked in, he asked me why I was there as if he'd never had an opportunity to learn anything about me beforehand. Once I started talking, he'd give me a fake smile, nod a few times as I spoke, then glance at Mary out of the corner of his eye as if to check whether she knew I was as whacked out as he thought I was. To be fair, my statement about why I'd come to see him probably sounded convoluted and hard to follow, but that's because it was. I couldn't verbalize a clear statement about why I needed his help because there was so much I didn't really know about what was wrong with me. What I ended up telling him was a rambling story with no definite beginning or direction because I didn't know it myself. Also, I looked fairly healthy on the outside, which might have indicated to him, albeit incorrectly, that I was pretty healthy on the inside, too. It was likely all of these things, but I couldn't help but wonder if my thick medical file, with all of the test results and doctor's notations from past visits, might have actually hindered my care rather than helped it. Who knows, maybe one or more doctors in my past had logged their opinion that my problems weren't in my body but in my head. If true, those words would be hard to overcome.

To be fair, if a doctor had doubted me, I could almost understand. I mean, who has so many seemingly unrelated symptoms that would appear, disappear, and then reappear again, maybe in a slightly different form? I could *almost* understand, but yet I couldn't because along the way, not one of them—not even *one*—ever stopped to take a moment to consult a book or a website or even to ask me more questions to help dig just a little deeper into the situation. Not one. In my experience, there was a common and clear arrogance among most in the traditional medical community. The clinics were willing to accept my payment but seemed much less interested in providing help. I realize that I didn't have a "cookie-cutter" ailment, but that shouldn't have mattered. I paid for their time and knowledge and deserved to have been carefully considered rather than been brushed aside.

Unfortunately, I didn't know of any other way to find answers that might help me other than to continue seeking the wisdom of traditional medical doctors. I'd heard great things about the genius discoveries and solutions at the renowned M. Clinic, and when I mentioned it to friends and neighbors, my confidence was bolstered by their own stories of success. So Mary scheduled an appointment for me, and we made plans to travel to Rochester for an evaluation. I was confident the doctors there would at least find my situation an intriguing challenge and wondered why I'd waited so long to get help from the best.

Chapter 13

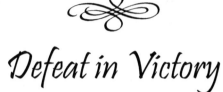

Defeat in Victory

Do you not know that those who run in a race all run, but only one receives the prize? Run in such a way that you may win. Everyone who competes in the games exercises self-control in all things. So they do it to obtain a perishable wreath, but we are imperishable.
1 Corinthians 9:24-25

At this point in my life, I was just hanging on. Sometimes it was by a thicker thread than others, but always doing my best, for whatever that was worth. My kids were growing up faster than I wanted, and I was fully aware that I wasn't able to be as active as they deserved. One of the most important parts of their lives for me was their involvement in sports. In this regard, all sports, but especially baseball, were important. Way before any of them was even born, I'd dreamed of the opportunity to develop their understanding of the game and their ability to play it. It started when my mom threw that grounder to me at seven years old, continued through my Little League experiences, and lingered still into the present.

I'd grown up amongst some pretty keen baseball enthusiasts. It was common for all the kids in the neighborhood to spend the afternoon playing in one of their big yards in town. When I wasn't playing there with the gang, I was throwing my baseball against the side of the barn, trying each time to hit a mark I'd made. My dream was to be a pitcher, so I'd throw the ball as fast as possible, then run after it as fast as I could, pick it up, sprint to my "pitcher's mound," and do it again. I did this so often that I started getting pretty good at it. After a while, I could hit that mark just about every time, even after sprinting back and forth. You might think I'd get sick of this and stop throwing, but I was obsessed. I loved baseball so much that I even chose to read a book about baseball great Sandy Kopeck. It was one of the only books I've ever read. It took me a long time to read, but I finished it. Boy, did I want to be him!

I'd done some pitching for my Little League team the previous year, and I'd been pretty good at it. I couldn't wait for the new season because I was finally at the age and had the ability to really prove my talent to my coaches, friends, and especially my mom. Unfortunately, when the season started, I discovered that the coach's son was a pitcher too. He was the apple of his father's eye—so big an apple his father could see little else. The coach had placed his son's two best friends on the team, and of course, they were pitchers too. To make a long story short, I was never given the opportunity to even set foot on the pitcher's mound that year. Not even in practice. The coach had no idea what I could do because he never gave me a chance to show him.

I know it's easy to overestimate one's ability when you're a kid, and most parents would do the same. My mom, though, wasn't like most moms: she was tough and fair and didn't romanticize or overstate anything. She was an ardent Cubs fan, and her own father had been a well-respected pitcher in his younger years, so she knew more than a little about the game. Even at age ninety-two, she'd tell you in a second how skillfully I pitched and how unfair it was that I was never given a chance to show it to the rest of the world.

I was heartbroken after that season, and surprisingly, it was just as painful in my adult years as it was then—maybe even more. I'd stayed with the team for a few more years, but my heart just wasn't in it. I regret that decision, though. I'm not sure if I was more disappointed because my dream had been squelched or because I'd given someone else so much control over my life. Maybe it was a little of both.

Defeat in Victory

After I gave baseball up, I started boxing, and as I've already shared, I did pretty well as a boxer. Boxing helped me fight back against the bullying I endured at school. Moreover, after that fight I lost but gave it everything I had to win the third round, I learned there can be a sense of victory in defeat.

Pretty soon, I had to quit boxing, too, because something happened to my hands. They would cramp up severely, and sometimes I couldn't even open them. This usually happened when I was at boxing practice or just after when I got home. After I stopped boxing, the frequency of my hand cramps diminished, then went away altogether. Still, I never found out what was behind it.

During high school, I competed in two sports: football and track. I didn't care for football that much, but my friends were all playing so I wanted to be part of it, too. The coaches made me a running back and a linebacker on the junior varsity team during my first two years. Then in my sophomore year, I was called up to play linebacker on the varsity team for the last few games of the season. It was fun to play with the older guys, and since it was a defensive position, I didn't need to memorize plays or study much of anything to be successful. It was mostly instinctive, and I was pretty good at that.

As a junior, I was on the varsity team all year, and this time I was expected to play both positions. The team needed a good running back, and they were looking to me to fill that role. Running backs obviously need to know the plays, which requires one to study and then memorize the playbook. Studying, however, was hard for me—even when sports were involved. The information just didn't seem to stick. So even though I tried to prepare, once game time came around, I wasn't ever confident that I knew what I was doing—which turned out to be the case: I didn't know what I was doing. No matter how hard I tried, I couldn't remember the plays.

It's one thing to feel embarrassed because you've goofed up, but it's another thing to be pointed out by the head coach in front of the rest of the players and all of the fans. I'm sure he was frustrated and wanted to emphasize to me that when I did the wrong thing, it affected everyone else on the team, and he probably thought that doing it so publicly would cause me to try a little harder. Even so, he didn't know that I was already doing the best I could. His words didn't just hurt me at that time but affected me for years to come in parts of my life other than just sports.

Over time, it seemed like the coaches just gave up on me. This was evident even during the pre-game routine. It was a tradition before every home game for the players to lie down on the gym floor for fifteen to twenty minutes in total peace and quiet. During this time, the coaches would walk around and stop by each player to say a few words of encouragement. It was meant to motivate and instill confidence in the players. When they came near me, however, they eventually continued on and didn't bother to stop and talk. I got my hopes up one day when I noticed one of the coaches approaching me. He bent down, said a few words, then suddenly stopped and looked a little closer at my face before standing up and moving on. He'd thought I was someone else. I'd always thought that the game was more important than me, and this made it abundantly clear.

You might wonder why I would stay in a situation that was so disheartening. To quit, though, would have been embarrassing because it would have made my failure even more evident than it probably already was. Also, because I'd done that in baseball, I knew I didn't want to allow these coaches to have that kind of power over me. The bullying I'd experienced as a child, along with the difficulties I'd experienced in school, had taught me determination. I wasn't a quitter, and I wasn't going to let anyone else win. That was evident in track.

The best thing about track is there is no playbook; it's all about ability and heart. It was something new for me, though, and while new things can sometimes be risky, I wasn't too concerned about failing. After all, I could run. So when the season rolled around, I was there and ready to go. I was intrigued by events such as the high jump, hurdles, and sprints and was motivated that the coach seemed to like me even from the start.

One of the first meets of the season was held on the indoor track in the gymnasium at the University of Wisconsin-Oshkosh. This meet was always very well-attended, and therefore the competition was tough. My coach signed me up for several track events and field events at that meet. Of all of them, I only remember the 440-yard race that day.

Defeat in Victory

I'd agreed to try the 440 when my coach had asked me about it a few days earlier. Now that the time was here, though, I was nervous. We'd have to circle the track two times rather than just once on this occasion since it was a smaller track than usual, which made the race seem more difficult. In addition, I was scheduled to run in the last heat, so I'd seen most of the other competitors run before it was my turn. As I headed toward the starting blocks, I promised not to embarrass myself by coming in last and resolved to just run hard so that didn't happen. I focused on the idea that this race was going to be about will: my will to control the situation and make it turn out in my favor. I was going to run harder and, therefore, faster than anyone else. It was as simple as that. I readied myself in the starting blocks.

Bang! The other runners shot out of the blocks, and I was in last place before taking even a few steps. At the end of the first corner, I was well behind the rest of the runners. I was still trying to figure out what they were doing that I wasn't when I rounded the second corner, and I was still just as far behind as ever. I lowered my head and reminded myself of my promise not to come in last. I pushed myself harder, taking longer and faster strides. Somewhere during the beginning of the second lap, I passed my first runner. The next one was in my sight, and it wasn't long before I ran by him too. Now my lungs were on fire. I was giving it all I had, and even though it felt like I wasn't speeding up, I wasn't slowing down either. The others in front of me must have been tiring, though, because I noticed that I was steadily closing the gap.

As I rounded the final curve and the finish line came into sight, I decided I'd rather burst my lungs and die than coast to the end. I dug deep and gave all I had left to pass the last two runners somehow and cross the finish line first in the heat. I immediately fell to all fours in complete exhaustion as the stadium started to spin around me, and I began dry-heaving. The coach ran over and helped me arch my back so I could breathe. After what felt like forever, he helped me up and led me off the track.

Through the mental haze of my exhaustion, I heard the announcer list the winners, and to my surprise, realized that I'd not only won my heat but the entire race! I collapsed into a chair as smiling teammates high-fived me, and other runners came over to offer their congratulations. My coach proudly gushed praise for my skill and determination, and even the spectators seemed to look at me with admiration.

With all these accolades, I should have felt proud about what I'd accomplished, but pride was not what filled my heart that day. Instead, I felt dread because I knew this performance had set a precedent for something I couldn't—or at least didn't want to—repeat. Sometimes even winning is losing, I realized.

All this is to say that organized sports had a big influence on my life. Unfortunately, most of my experiences with it were negative, so as my children approached their various ages of participation, I was determined to ensure that their involvement in athletics would be more rewarding than mine. I couldn't wait for opportunities when I could coach them on proper techniques, have conversations with them about the game, and watch them play. Now that this time had come, one of my greatest hopes was that I would be healthy enough to be involved with them during the process. The second was that they'd have more success with it than me.

The first stop on the journey was T-ball. It didn't take long to conclude that you can't really count it as a sport, but instead just a bunch of kids throwing a ball around to a bunch of other kids trying to catch it—none with very much success. Honestly, given my lofty dreams, it was painful to watch. Still, I guess they had to start somewhere. I was sure my children would catch on quickly, though—especially with my experience and guidance. So I tried to be enthusiastic and encouraging, and slowly but surely, the little tykes increased their control and attention so that they were more focused on the action on the diamond than the dandelions growing from it.

Because of my vow to be involved in my children's athletic endeavors, I jumped at the chance to take a coaching role when one was available. The sport I felt most passionate about and most comfortable with was baseball, so that was where I was most involved. I tried to maintain the impartiality I'd not been shown when I was a kid so that every child would feel valued on the team, but I was mostly there for my children. Not just because I wanted each of them to have the best chance for success but because, at that point in my life, I truly felt that I was dying. It seemed like it wouldn't be long that same year, or maybe that year or sometime in the near future that I would get one last glimpse of my children doing what I'd so loved to do. I couldn't have given you an estimate of how long I had left, but I felt certain that my days on this earth were quite limited.

I had begun to coach my oldest son, Joe, from his earliest baseball days. By his seventh-grade year, however, I was really sick, really tired, and seemed to have more things going wrong than ever before.

A few months before that season started, I began to experience quivers in my back, especially around my shoulders. I also began to notice the throb of my heartbeat pounding through my entire body. I don't mean I could just *kind* of notice the lub-dub, lub-dub rhythm—I mean, I could *intensely* feel it. Since the symptoms I was having seemed closely linked to my heart, I went against my better judgment and made an appointment to see a doctor. Maybe I was having a heart attack, or perhaps my blood pressure was really high, both instances that one didn't want to wait around to think about.

Typically, I'd take some time to strategically plan which doctor or clinic to visit since I'd already seen so many local ones and hadn't felt that any of them had given me the consideration or respect needed because of my complicated past. The gravity of this situation, however, seemed to lessen the necessity of such deep thought about the matter. I felt sure this time, no doctor would just send me off with a pat on the back and a few encouraging words. There could be nothing else but a serious issue, after all.

So, after Mary said a prayer for guidance (something she'd recently started to do with the hope that God would bring us to someone just right for the situation), she picked a doctor, gave the clinic a call, and scheduled an appointment. As we'd done so many times before, we both hoped that this doctor would realize something no one else had considered and that this visit would somehow lead us to answers that would explain all of my other health challenges.

We shouldn't have been surprised, but we were dismayed. The doctor we saw that day had ". . . never before in his whole life heard of such a thing." According to him, I was simply suffering from "significant body awareness" but apparently was otherwise just fine. At that time, it seemed like that was just about the most idiotic diagnosis I'd ever heard. *Significant body awareness...?* I could only shake my head as I left the clinic that day. Not only did this appointment add to my frustration, but it would also result in one more report in my file that would make me look nuts. Once more, I was without any help and now had even less faith in the medical community's desire or ability to help me. Worst of all, my symptoms really scared me.

Chapter 14

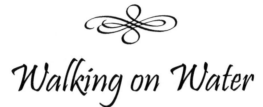

Walking on Water

And He said, "Come!" And Peter got out of the boat and walked on the water, and came toward Jesus. But seeing the wind, he became frightened, and when he began to sink, he cried out, saying, "Lord, save me!"

Matthew 14:29-30

Everything we'd heard about the M. Clinic was positive. "They'll get to the bottom of it," a neighbor assured us. Others smiled and nodded when we mentioned our upcoming appointment, seemingly assured that this would be the end of our troubles. Unfortunately, I wasn't easily convinced and instead felt that my future was almost certainly short and very bleak. Most of the time until now I'd tried to keep my despair to myself, but I'd physically and emotionally reached rock bottom and now felt it was time for me to share what I saw as my likely demise with them.

I called the kids into the bedroom one day as I lay there exhausted as usual. They probably came in expecting me to ask them to help relieve some of my physical discomforts: to sit on my chest or walk on my back in an attempt to lessen my indigestion or to take turns digging their nails into my feet to ease those aches and pains. This time though was about emotional rather than physical relief. I wanted them to know how serious I believed my situation to be; to know that barring some type of drastic revelation, I wouldn't be around any longer. I just didn't want it to be a huge shock to them when it occurred.

After I bluntly explained my predicament, the room became very quiet as tears began to flow and the kids wrapped their arms around me. Mary, who had fiercely opposed my plan to share this information with the children, did her best to remain optimistic and encouraging. Nonetheless, her words mostly fell on deaf ears. It was a terrible time for all of us. I could feel my life slipping away.

My words and actions at that time may seem melodramatic, but a closer look at my life during that time reflects how dire my situation had become. I was able to tolerate only two types of food: red meat and rice. As a result, my weight had plummeted to about 150 pounds from the robust 200 pounds I had weighed only six months earlier. My cheeks were gaunt, my body emaciated, and my pallor ashen. It was difficult for me to walk even thirty feet without being exhausted. In addition, I was experiencing an incredible number of symptoms that varied inexplicably in duration and intensity, including:

- Back muscle quivers
- Food allergies and intolerances
- Nutrition deficiency
- Back pain
- Groin and leg pain
- Irregular neural sensations
- Blisters and sores
- Head fog
- Periodic loss of vision
- Body shocks
- Head pain
- Persistent pneumonia
- Exploding head syndrome
- Burning feet
- Heartburn
- Severe depression
- Chest pain
- Hematuria (blood in urine)
- Tingling feet
- Constipation
- Hemorrhoids
- Urination pain
- Diarrhea
- Inability to urinate
- Ulcerative colitis
- Whole-body soreness

- Leg cramps
- Very low blood pressure
- Extreme fatigue
- Leg pain
- Whole-body trembling
- Eye pressure
- Lower leg nodules
- Whole-body numbness
- Facial numbness
- Neck pain

Before leaving for the M. Clinic, I had a strong desire to play golf one more time, just in case it might be my last. I remember standing by the tee box of one of the holes, looking out at the beautiful fields. I saw the greens and browns of God's splendor and was simply overwhelmed by it all. Tears began to flow down my face as I took in great gulps of His clean, fresh air. It wasn't that I'd never noticed those things before nor given thanks to Him for them, but it was at that moment likely due to my intense grief.

I'd been playing golf consistently throughout my health crisis simply because it helped me feel at least somewhat normal, even though it wasn't especially fun or rewarding. There was so little about how I now lived that matched the lifestyles of my friends or even neighbors because of the physical and dietary situations that I constantly needed to maneuver around. My days were neither simple nor carefree like theirs at least appeared to be. So I fought to continue faking normalcy by way of eighteen holes of golf, but even that was now almost unbearable.

The appointment at the clinic was set for a Monday morning in early August. We were told that we were lucky to get in as quickly as we had, so we were extremely thankful about that and hoped it was a sign that good things were ahead. The school year hadn't yet begun, so it wasn't hard for Mary or the kids to get away for a week. We found a nice hotel not too far away, and the kids were excited about the opportunity to swim and explore there for several days. We checked in the night before, rested well, and headed to the clinic together for my first appointment on Monday morning.

I was scheduled first to meet with an allergist. I'd been "assigned" to him since his specialty seemed most closely aligned with my main concern. He would be the one to take my history and schedule further appointments with other specialists if needed. I took the opportunity seriously and wanted to be sure to tell every pertinent detail. It was a thorough, passionate explanation of all I could think of that might be relevant. When I was done, the physician didn't seem very moved, had no significant solution, and did what I imagine he did for every other patient he saw: scheduled a few blood tests and made some additional appointments. I was scheduled to see a dyslexia specialist, a dietician, and a gastroenterologist. As we left his exam room, Mary and I exchanged a well-worn look of exasperation. We both recognized that despite his employment at this well-renowned clinic, this specialist seemed just as stoic and uninformed as what we'd experienced locally. Still, we tried to remain hopeful that someone we'd encounter during our time here would uncover something that would be helpful. *Anything.* This was M. Clinic, after all! People came here from all over the world looking for, and often finding cures for all kinds of ailments—or so we were told.

My additional appointments weren't until the next day, so we returned to the hotel and gave the kids some time in the pool. It was hard to mirror their enthusiasm for this experience, though, because the day hadn't felt very successful and we knew the stakes were high. We returned to the clinic on Tuesday, curious about how input from the dyslexia specialist and dietician would prove helpful. An hour later, we left the office of the dyslexia specialist after having been reminded that dyslexia was a difficult issue with no cure; a condition that could only be partially remediated and one in which an individual's best hope was to learn coping strategies that might alleviate the effects of the disability. So far, it was Strike Two.

We turned our attention to the appointment with the dietician. This one was promising. We were certain to learn something new here about the latest nutrition information and how food intake could be adjusted to help digestion and alter my body's unusual reaction to it. We were barely settled into our seats for our appointment when the woman who introduced herself as the dietician invited us to share with her what would constitute my typical day's diet. It was pretty easy for me to explain—and I didn't have to worry about forgetting anything—because there were so few foods to include. I told her that I started the day with a piece of salmon, had some type of red meat and rice for lunch, and finished my day with a meal of either red meat or chicken and a potato. I emphasized that I was not eating any dairy, fruit, vegetables, and very few grains because my body didn't seem able to tolerate them.

The dietician scribbled my words quickly upon her notebook as I spoke. When I was finished, she quickly skimmed her notes to select key bits of information she wanted to touch upon. Her first comment was that my body definitely needed a greater variety of nutrients and that since some of the most important ones were found in vegetables, it was essential that I make them part of my diet. Of course, I already knew this and would have loved to do so. My experience, however, had been that my body reacted in strange and uncomfortable ways after eating vegetables, which had suggested to me that I was allergic to them and therefore caused me to believe that I should avoid them.

The dietician smiled politely and allowed me to finish my thoughts about the subject, then told me that the symptoms I had shared simply weren't what would occur if I was having an allergic response. Food allergy symptoms, she emphasized, included breathing difficulties, hives, and diarrhea that occurred within twelve hours of exposure to the allergen rather than the body tingling, neck stiffness, and brain fog I'd experienced, sometimes as long as forty-eight hours after I ate. I tried to explain the theory of delayed allergic responses that Mary and I had read about during her investigations of the subject but was told that this condition simply wasn't accurate.

When an expert at the M. Clinic tells you that you are wrong about something, there's not much you can do other than to sit back, shut your mouth, and nod your head as if you are thankful for every morsel of insight they are feeding you. It doesn't mean, though, you agree with it or that you're happy about having to listen to it, which we weren't. I wonder if the dietician thought our now docile demeanors meant that she'd convinced us of the truth or if she recognized our reality: that we'd simply turned our arguments inward and weren't really listening to any of her advice about how to diversify my diet according to the food pyramid that was the ultimate healthy eating guide at that time—because we knew it wouldn't work for me. When our appointment was finally over, we smiled and thanked the dietician, then walked out the door and sighed. Strike Three.

To say that things hadn't worked out as we'd hoped would be an understatement. Still, we hoped that tomorrow's appointment with the gastroenterologist would be helpful and that the top-notch physicians here would have a remedy that might, at least slightly, take the edge off my condition. So on Wednesday morning, we packed our bags in the car since we'd be leaving for home right after the appointment and headed back to the clinic one more time. We entered through the now-familiar glass and marble entranceway with less confidence but just as much hope as we'd felt that first time several days earlier. The elevator ride to the upper floors of the clinic was exciting for the kids, and the view through the large glass panels in the waiting room was certainly impressive for all of us. We registered, took a seat in the waiting room, and made small talk as if this appointment wasn't the big deal that it was. When I was finally called into the exam room for my appointment, I took a deep breath and said a quick prayer. When I returned to this spot in an hour's time, would I be a changed man? Would I finally have some hope?

The wait in the exam room felt longer than usual, but eventually, a young woman and a medical student in training knocked on the door and entered. Her demeanor was pleasant but curt, and it was clear that she was all business. She told me that she'd read the notes provided by the specialist I'd seen several days earlier, so I didn't need to recount my history for her. Her recommendation was that since I'd been diagnosed with ulcerative colitis, it was imperative that I take the medication that had been prescribed for me and that there wasn't anything else she could do. When I emphasized to her that my body didn't seem to tolerate it very well, she suggested that I try a different type of medication. I explained that I'd already done that but that all medications seemed to negatively and significantly bother me after a while, so I'd found no other solution than to stop taking them. Upon hearing this news, her patience, which had seemed short even upon entering the room, seemed even more abbreviated. She looked me in the eye and told me clearly and plainly that I had two options for care: take the medication by mouth or have it inserted in the other end. There was nothing else that could be done. It wasn't hard to see that there was no point in trying, once again, to clarify my situation. She wasn't interested in it and had nothing more to add. I probably mumbled some kind of response as she mechanically shook my hand and turned to leave the room, but I don't remember much about it. We exited the room, gathered the kids from the waiting area, and rode the elevator silently down to the main floor. With heavy hearts, we found the car, piled in, and began our long drive home.

Several hours on the road provided plenty of time to think about what a disappointment the last few days had been. We were leaving with absolutely no new information and a whole lot less hope. None of these fancy, renowned doctors had any "eureka" revelations, and to be honest, most didn't even seem to care. I guess that's only natural when thousands of sick people flood through the doors day after day. To them, I'd just been one more unhealthy guy to examine, but to me, they'd been my ultimate hope.

We had given it our best shot. If the specialists at the M. Clinic had no idea, then who would? I grimly faced the reality that I may have mere weeks left, and I had just spent thousands of dollars that could have helped my family pay for my funeral and burial costs. I was overcome with sadness and cried all the way home. I was really going to miss my family.

When I was a child, I would sometimes challenge myself to walk all the way across a room with my eyes closed. I would take a good, long look at my surroundings, then close my eyes and start to move. My goal was to see how far I could get without putting out my hands. The plan was to walk slowly but confidently, without stretching out my hands until I was certain I was at the wall on the other side of the room. More times than not, I would stop, open my eyes and find out I had only crept about halfway. In those times, I knew, before opening my eyes, I could have gone further. I didn't have the faith necessary to trust what I knew to be true.

I recalled this scenario within a few days of my return from the M. Clinic and it ultimately gave me the hope I needed to change the course of my life. Until now, I'd come to accept that my end was near, and there was nothing left to do but submit to it. My recollection, however, revealed a different course. Instead of just giving in and giving up, I could give my condition—my pain and my dismal future—to God. I could choose to have faith that everything was in His hands. Instead of opening my eyes to take control of where I was going, like when I was a child, I could keep them closed and let faith in God guide me instead. The apostle Peter began to sink when he began to consider the giant waves and terrible storm around him instead of trusting Jesus to keep him safe (see Matthew 14:29-30), and I'd been doing the same.

It was the easiest thing in the world to say I believed in God. I'd been doing it all my life. I'd told my children, my siblings, my co-workers, and my neighbors about how much I loved God. I read the Bible, went to church, and even led Bible studies. Still, I was almost completely devoid of what I needed the most: true faith.

I closed my eyes and pleaded with God for Him to give me another chance. I told Him I knew of His love, His power, and His desire for me to have comfort and contentment. I prayed for understanding about why He was allowing me to remain sick and asked Him to give me a reprieve if it was His will. Also, I told Him that I trusted Him to do what He needed to do with my life to fulfill His will and that no matter what happened, I'd serve Him and remain faithful to Him.

As I finished my prayer, I remembered that every once in a while, as a kid, I was able to walk across an entire room with my eyes closed. It took courage, patience, persistence, and, most of all, faith. When I'd accomplished my feat through faith so many years ago, I felt like a champion. I felt the same way again today.

Chapter 15

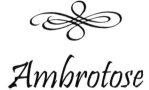

Ambrotose

One day He was teaching, and there were some Pharisees and teachers of the Law sitting there who had come from every village of Galilee and Judea, and from Jerusalem; and the power of the Lord was present for Him to perform healing.
Luke 5:17

Six days after returning from the M. Clinic, a co-worker told me about a health presentation scheduled after work hours at the plant. She knew of my health struggles and thought I'd be interested in hearing about something she thought might help. To be sure, the last thing I wanted to do was to stay an hour later at work to listen to anything, let alone a health presentation. I wasn't even certain about the topic. Nevertheless, to show appreciation for my colleague's concern for me, I felt obligated to stay.

When I arrived in the conference room, about ten other staff were already seated near the front. I was surprised when I saw the presenter because I recognized her as someone I'd worked with for several years. Her name was Vicki, and I'd actually gone to high school with her, as well.

I can't recall the details of the presentation partly because I didn't pay very close attention to it; I was exhausted from the shift I'd just completed. In addition, I didn't really think she'd be able to help me. I remember, however, that she began by talking about the importance of eating healthy food, then discussed how much of today's food supply is nutritionally deficient. It soon dawned on me that this was a sales pitch about nutritional supplements created by a company called Mannatech. The feature item was called Ambrotose, and according to the presenter, it was a miraculous product.

When the presentation was over, I approached Vicki. I am sure she could see how very physically challenged I was at the time, but I still said, "You know I am very, very sick."

Without a pause, she slugged me playfully in the arm and replied, "Don't worry about it. You'll be fine."

I repeated, "You don't understand. I am very, very sick." I wanted her to understand that because of my serious condition, I wasn't interested in any flippant sales promises. Still, despite my obvious frailty and melancholy tone, her response was incredibly upbeat and confident. She grabbed my arm, looked me square in the eye, and repeated firmly, "Don't worry about it. You'll be fine."

For some reason, her words—and the confident tone in which she spoke them—were the shot of hope I so desperately needed. I had no idea how she could look at me and, in all sincerity and boldness, say those words: "You'll be fine." I was gaunt, pale, and listless. Still, she was positive and enthusiastic. I was pretty sure she was just ignoring the obvious in order to make a sale, but maybe, just maybe, she really meant it.

What I didn't yet understand was Vicki's personal experience with Ambrotose. She'd used it to resolve a serious health crisis of her own. She told me it had helped her and many others in ways that were almost unbelievable. I was intrigued by her story and even more impressed when I heard that Mannatech, the company that created this amazing product, was vocally Christian in their words and deeds.

Further drawing my interest was the fact that third-party clinical trials had shown Ambrotose to provide a wide array of health benefits, including neurological support and improved function of all body organs, with special emphasis on gastrointestinal health. I was told this resulted from plant saccharides called glyconutrients in the supplement that supported cell-to-cell communication. She told me that all I needed to do was liberally ingest the powder several times a day and that within the week, I'd see a noticeable improvement in my health.

Of course, I was skeptical. I had a hard time believing anything—or anyone—could help me at this point. Nevertheless, I reckoned I had nothing to lose except the money it was going to cost me for the supplements. So when Vicki told me that I could get my money back after sixty days if I wasn't happy with the product, nothing could hold me back from trying it.

As soon as the product arrived, I began to do exactly what she'd suggested: I took a scoop of Ambrotose powder twice a day. For the first couple of days, I didn't notice any difference. On the third day, I thought I might be feeling a little better, but I wasn't sure if it was just because I was thinking so much about it or if it was really happening. By the fourth day, though, I was sure of its effect because I began to feel significantly better. By the end of the week, I had more energy than I'd had in a long time—maybe as much as three times what I'd been experiencing. I still felt pretty weak, but for the first time in a long time, I didn't feel as though I was knocking on death's door. That in itself was worth getting on my knees and thanking God for because He had not only sent me my acquaintance, who advocated the Ambrotose, but also my colleague at work who'd persuaded me to attend the presentation.

I continued taking the Ambrotose powder liberally for the next several weeks. Each week, my energy increased. Ironically, I didn't measure Ambrotose's effect upon me by the increase in energy I felt but instead by the decrease in toxicity I experienced after having taken it for even this short period of time. It amazed me that this one rather unassuming product had done so much for me so quickly. Furthermore, I was astounded that it had come to me in what seemed to be my last days. It was suddenly clear that God's divine intervention had saved my life. I don't know why He had waited so long—almost to the point of what I felt was my certain impending death—but He had. I'd heard that God's timing is perfect, and even though I wasn't very excited about it at the time, I reluctantly knew this was true.

Although I still had a lot of physical issues, the Ambrotose had helped me considerably, which relieved some of the pressure in our home. During the next few months, I was able to tolerate a greater variety of foods and slowly began to regain the weight I'd lost. My improved physical health led to increased optimism and relief in our home, which was desperately needed.

My body had finally taken at least one step in the right direction, which should have made me happy. Still, as much as I hate to admit it, there was a part of me that secretly wished God hadn't intervened to improve my health. I'd mentally prepared myself for death, which would have enabled me to escape what was so often such a miserable existence. After several months passed and my improvements had somewhat plateaued, I pondered why God had chosen to keep me here on Earth, especially since it didn't seem like the Ambrotose alone was going to fix all of my problems. What was He trying to teach me, and why did it all have to be so hard? It was hard not to be at least a little ungrateful since I was still suffering in so many ways.

It was during this time that I began to recall an experience I'd had when I was about eleven or twelve years old. It was a silly debate with my older sister, Tina, about whether or not I needed food. Obviously, I knew that a body needs food for its physical survival, but in this debate with Tina, I was pushing the idea that I didn't have an *emotional* need for food. It was clear that day and so many afterward that my stance about food couldn't have been more wrong! Food is much more than physical sustenance and has very significant social and emotional components. Food is often the centerpiece of gatherings during holidays, family reunions, church functions, work parties, birthdays, etc. Consider also the anticipation that is so common with any upcoming Thanksgiving meal or Independence Day barbeque. Now think about what it would be like if these things led to feelings of isolation and deprivation instead of unity and joy. In my case, social functions were experiences to endure rather than to enjoy. Furthermore, although I couldn't eat the food, I still had to smell the delicious aroma and watch everyone around me eating and drinking and connecting with each other in ways only those who are fully immersed in the experience can do. Sometimes it was unbearable, and I had to leave the building altogether. At other times, I was able to prepare myself for the disappointment and loneliness I would almost definitely face so that I could make it through without overwhelming discomfort. Occasionally someone would make a comment about my dour expression or question why I'd packed myself a plain chicken breast and a bit of rice as if I had chosen to bring it from home because it was just too good to pass up. On the rare occasion that I gave into temptation and allowed myself even a small bite of one or more of the delicious, "dangerous" items someone was serving. I would always pay the price later with stomach cramps, diarrhea, body aches, or some other weird symptom. It was *never* worth it. So Tina was right—I *do* need food—more than I ever could have imagined!

Throughout the next year, I kept in touch with Vicki, and she offered many suggestions to try to help me. She talked to me about liver and colon cleanses and other things that people found to be quite helpful in managing their health. Still, other than adding in some Optimal Support Supplements from Mannatech, anything I tried either didn't have any effect upon me or, worse yet, caused me to feel even more discomfort. Mary also continued to research options, which led to me trying colon hydrotherapy, coffee enemas, infrared saunas, acupuncture, and Epsom salt baths. Some of these helped a little, but none made such a difference that I knew I was on the right track. These options were just Band-Aids—never a complete solution.

I continued to spend a great deal of time on my knees praying, begging, and wondering. Most of all, though, I was learning. I was learning to fall deeply in love with my Father. I was also recognizing that I needed to talk with Him not only when I was feeling lousy but on those days and in those moments when I was feeling better too. I just needed to talk with Him, as one would to a friend, but I also needed to show Him gratitude. This understanding developed slowly but really blossomed after I'd found success with Mannatech and recognized His role in bringing me to it. At this point, I began to pray more deeply and more often, mostly because it seemed like this was the first time He had reached down to help me. Of course, this wasn't true because it was actually the first time that I'd really, with all my being, reached up to Him.

After a while, however, despite the initial relief I'd experienced with the Ambrotose, my improvement began to plateau. I'd always worried it wouldn't be a long-term solution, and unfortunately, it was now starting to prove true. The success it had brought, however, opened a new door for me because now that I'd personally experienced support from a natural remedy,

Mary and I had other additional paths to explore outside of those provided through Western Medicine.

One of the first options we chose was a naturopath in Madison, which was a little more than an hour southwest of us. Doctor Aaron was a young, enthusiastic, intelligent Christian man who had recently started his own practice. At that time, his naturopathic clinic was one of very few in the entire state. From the very first moment I met him, it was clear that this was the place for me. The interest he took in me and my health challenges was incredible compared to what I had experienced in so many allopathic clinics before him. He spent most of one whole hour just listening to me on that first day. He never rushed me or passed judgment about anything I told him. He didn't smirk at me contemptuously, and he didn't ever suggest he knew what the matter was—or wasn't.

At each appointment, he tried a little of this and a little of that and carefully documented any success—or results that didn't seem to be as successful as we'd hoped. We tried supplements, electrotherapy, and even prayed together. Then, we'd wait a week or two to observe the treatment outcomes and meet again to revise the protocol. One of Doctor Aaron's suggestions was to have blood drawn to check the levels of toxins in my body. Since I worked at a plastics thermoforming plant, he believed there was a likelihood the melted plastics in the air around me at work may be causing these issues. I'd often wondered the same thing, but after having been assured by the company that their safety protocols were appropriate (and seeing considerable documentation that seemed to prove it), I'd always pushed such concerns to the back of my mind.

When the test results came back, however, Doctor Aaron noticed some elevated levels that concerned him, so he suggested I see a toxicologist to help identify what could be done to mitigate them. The nearest toxicologist who would meet with patients (who apparently just did research) was a specialist near Chicago. Mary wasted no time in setting up the appointment. We were so excited to finally have uncovered an issue that seemed to really hold some promise for better health.

On the day of the appointment, we left home before dawn so we'd be sure to get to the facility on time. When we checked in, the receptionist seemed confused about why we were there and who we were to see. Eventually, she asked us to take a seat in the waiting room. We weren't sure if that meant she had clarified the issue or if she needed more time without us being within earshot as she tried to resolve it. We waited nervously for a long time until, finally, a nurse appeared and called my name. We followed her through a tangle of hallways to a small room that looked more like a well-used closet than a consultation room. It was spacious enough but didn't seem to be the kind of place people were seen in on a regular basis. No problem, I thought, and we assured each other with a mutual glance that this was going to be epic; this was the moment that would finally change everything.

When the toxicologist arrived, he had an air of someone who had been interrupted from doing something he enjoyed to do something he did not enjoy. He was disheveled and a little on edge, as if he were impatient to return to more important matters. He curtly asked why we had come. We told him our story and handed him a copy of the toxicology report we had brought with us. He took his glasses out of his pocket and glanced at the report, flipping through the pages rather quickly. He then lifted his glasses to rest on his forehead to address us. Barely looking us in the eye, the toxicologist matter-of-factly informed us the elevated levels weren't really cause for concern. Although the levels looked high to us, he insisted they really weren't indicative of anything significant and were nothing about which to be alarmed. He said this in a dry, emotionless way that displayed not even the slightest bit of empathy. Maybe he thought he was giving us good news with this announcement as if his news would give us relief, but it didn't. Instead, it was not at all a relief but was a complete and utter disappointment and a scenario with which we were all too familiar. Since it seemed like no more than five minutes had passed from the time of his arrival to the time of his pronouncement, we tried to pull some more information from the man—to give him greater detail about my situation in an attempt to get him to consider the situation more deeply and perhaps then come to a different conclusion. Apparently, however, he didn't have anything more to say, and almost before I could have imagined, he shook my hand and exited the room. Somewhat stunned, we dejectedly did the same. It was difficult to resist the urge to slam the door behind us in disgust. We had three hours in the car on the way home to kick ourselves for even considering consulting anyone in the Western medical field again.

Chapter 16

Western Let Down

*Heal me, LORD, and I will be healed; save me
and I will be saved, for You are my praise.*
Jeremiah 17:14

In pain and despair, I watched my health deteriorate slowly and steadily to its lowest point. Each day was worse than its predecessor, although once in a while, I was blessed with one that was only equally as difficult as the one before. This period was the darkest time in my life. I lived in a constant state of extreme exhaustion and intense depression, battling to provide and be present as a father and husband. I'd go through the motions with as much energy as I could muster, but inwardly I'd started to focus more on death than life as my rollercoaster ride continued.

From the time I woke each morning, I felt only disappointment. First, because I'd awoken at all, and second because I quickly realized all over again that I'd have to get through another twenty-four hours without relief and options for support. I'd looked far and wide and had tried all kinds of options, but every single time I'd come to a dead end. Now there seemed nowhere else to turn. All of the supplements and treatments and specialists simply weren't able to help me. To make matters worse, I knew that as miserable as I was today, it would only be worse tomorrow. How would I ever be able to cope next week or next month or next year? I was miserable and completely overwhelmed.

When my alarm shrieked at 5:30 a.m. every morning, I spent the first twenty minutes of awareness lying there, cursing the day I was born. Sometimes I cried, and others, I just gritted my teeth and contemplated how I was going to deal with today's pain. The discomfort in my chest, back, feet, leg, groin, stomach, shoulder, and neck pain (all of which were most intense on the left side of my body for some reason) was different than it would be later in the day when I was somewhat distracted by my work. It was different from how I'd feel toward the end of my physically demanding eight hours on the job, but all hours of my day were difficult. Needless to say, it took me a while to get out of bed. It was also hard for me to get moving because once I was upright, dizziness, head fog, and pressure behind my eyes reappeared, which required even more resolve.

Despite how I felt, I tried to be thankful for the good things in my life. The kids were well-behaved and were getting good grades. Julia was on the swim team and also played school and travel team volleyball. Joe and Stephen played baseball, basketball, and football. Many weekday afternoons and evenings—and often both days of most weekends—were spent watching one child or more at a game or meet. In addition to loving them, I was extremely proud of them and thoroughly enjoyed watching them participate in their activities. I followed them wherever they went as often as I could. By this point, however, staying involved was getting near impossible, which added to the overall frustration I felt about my life.

Still, I fought to stay involved with them, and on the weekends when they weren't playing in a tournament or I wasn't completely wiped out, I would take the boys to the park to hit pop-ups and grounders or play catch with them at home. I coached one or both of their teams in baseball for a few years, even though I felt like death warmed up the entire time. Unfortunately, the worst thing I did the entire time was lose my patience about their apparent lack of desire to improve. They just wouldn't commit to the drills and repetitions I suggested and rarely sought my advice about how to play better defense, improve at the plate, or run a better route. I was driven to make them the players the coaches wouldn't overlook as I had been. When they were, I drove them even harder, ironically reflecting the unforgiving coaches I'd experienced myself. The difference in attitudes led to countless arguments and hurtful words from all parties, which continue to impact our relationships today.

In addition to driving them too hard, I tend to speak bluntly, which means that a lot of the time, my actions and words may have overwhelmed my kids (I know Mary thinks they did). Perhaps if I'd taken a different approach, I could have been more successful in influencing them. Of course, being raised by a mom who was tough-as-nails herself probably didn't help, either. Still, as I look back, I don't see how I could have interacted with my children in any other way. I was fighting for survival and had to be extremely tough on myself every single moment just to make it through the day. If I'd let my guard down for even a second, I'd be crushed. I believe I unconsciously felt I had to teach my children to approach life in the same way and that by pushing and speaking to them in such ways, I could inoculate them against the hard knocks of the world.

During this time, my relationship with Mary certainly wasn't thriving, but because of the seriousness of my condition, neither of us was in a position to do much about it. We both were living with a lot of pain. Mine has been pretty well documented here, but she had a great deal of it, too. Her job was overwhelming, as were the demands upon her (both spoken and unspoken) to bring me relief from my misery and discomfort. She was frustrated by our inability to build our savings since so much money was constantly being spent to find remedies or specialists to help me. In addition, I wasn't a very supportive or positive partner. My attitude and words frequently had a negative effect on the household, and I usually didn't have the energy or interest to participate in family activities, so she was left to do them all herself—or just not do them at all. Above all, she was scared that I might not even survive the next six months. Ironically what was tearing us apart was also holding us together. Her worry for me probably kept us together through a situation where it wouldn't have if I had been healthier. On the other hand, if I'd been healthier, maybe we wouldn't have been in that situation altogether.

I knew Mary wasn't happy, and although it was hard to know how to make things better, I tried to give her small joys when I could. Once in a while, I'd bring her flowers or something else from the store, but one of her favorite pleasures was a drive in the country—especially in the summer and fall. We'd take a road less traveled out of town and continue for about an hour, then make our way back. Late morning or early afternoon drives in the sunshine once a month or so were peaceful and refreshing for both of us. It was one of our only indulgences that we both enjoyed and could do together, but we did little else because I really just wanted to be at home in bed every chance I could get. Sleep had become one of my few escapes.

Every year as the summer ended, I dreaded the arrival of colder weather because of the increased discomfort that always came with it. One symptom, in particular, was an amplified discomfort in the ever-present pain in my chest. Eventually, it was difficult and painful to breathe, and breathing was accompanied by phlegm and cough. Before long, I had chills, a sore throat, and a low-grade fever. For most, this might mean a trip to the doctor for some antibiotics and some form of pain relief, but since my body doesn't tolerate medicine and it seemed unlikely that there would be any other treatment plan, there seemed to be no point. I was so physically and mentally broken at this point that I didn't just cry about my problems at home—I cried about them everywhere. I was also on my knees praying several times a day.

Sometimes at work, the pain was so severe that I could hardly breathe. One afternoon, after struggling to breathe for most of the day, I realized I was actually gasping for air and began to panic. My mind screamed, *Am I going to die? Is this it?* I just wasn't able to get the air I needed. My reaction at that point surprised me because I realized then and there that I really didn't want to live.

In the past, I'd contemplated the relief that dying would bring, so it puzzled me that I was now so concerned about it. If I passed away right here, how would the kids and my wife take the news? I was devastated to think that I'd be unable to say goodbye to them and to so many other people that I loved. I felt so sad to do this to my dear, precious Mary. For some bizarre reason, in the midst of the pain and panic, I also considered how embarrassing it would be to die at work. I never wanted anyone to see me in a position of weakness. Still, there I was, on the brink of dying, worrying about what people might think.

A friend of mine working nearby noticed me struggling and helped me to the plant manager's office. The manager was on the phone as I stumbled through the doorway, and he could see I was gasping for air. Since I was still standing, however, I guess he wasn't about to put his boss on hold until I hit the floor and turned blue. When he eventually finished his conversation, my breathing was somewhat better. He took a few minutes to talk with me and then excused me for the rest of the day.

Despite my lack of confidence in western medicine, I was both scared enough and felt obligated enough (since I'd been given the rest of the day off from work, after all) to drive to the emergency room at the nearest hospital on the other side of town. I wish I could say the medical professionals there surprised me with their wisdom and concern, but they didn't. They offered no theories or treatment. Whatever had caused me to believe I was knocking on death's door was a mystery. My only relief at the time was that Mary had arrived to be with me. If I were going to die, at least I would be able to say goodbye.

Chapter 17

Embedded and Undetectable

*Be devoted to one another in brotherly love;
give preference to one another in honor, not
lagging behind in diligence, fervent in spirit,
serving the Lord; rejoicing in hope, persevering
in tribulation, devoted to prayer, contributing to
the needs of the saints, practicing hospitality.*
Romans 12:10-13

A few years after high school, I joined a golf league with my friends. We'd play every Tuesday during the summer months, which soon became the highlight of my work week. Once I became so sick, however, golf was little more than another occasion just to try to endure. I had to use the same attitude to continue participating in golf that I'd done with work: If I let discomfort stop me today, there was little to prevent me from doing so again tomorrow, and the next day, and the next, and so on indefinitely. Also, what else was there if I let my body stop me from work and play?

One day while I was golfing, the first indication of a serious new symptom arrived as an unusual tightness in my arms. I was teeing off on the third hole when I suddenly felt a shattering sensation in my chest, a pattern of pain that spread like the splintering of a windshield hit just right by a large stone. I flinched, gasped, and took a moment to get my breath. As I indicated earlier, I don't like others to know about my physical struggles, so as frightening as the situation was for me, I continued playing and eventually finished the round as if nothing had happened. Once I got into my car, however, and began to drive away from the course, I began to sob. My body was breaking down bit by bit, and it seemed that there was nothing I could do about it.

When I got home, Mary and I discussed the incident and tried to decide what to do. If I went to the emergency room, the doctors would likely have no idea what was causing the discomfort and send me off the same as when I'd arrived, except for a few hundred dollars poorer. Even so, pain in one's chest isn't something to ignore, so it soon was clear that it was the right choice.

To make a long story short, the doctor on call that day had never heard of anything like this. My vitals were taken, and everything seemed to be working fine. Perhaps just to feel like he had done something, the doctor gave me an IV. As I lay there receiving the saline drip, I began to experience a surprising overall sense of well-being. My chest muscles relaxed, and my discomfort diminished. When the nurse checked in on me, I mentioned this to her. She smiled, rechecked my vitals, and left the room without much of a response. Even the doctor, who looked in on me once the IV drip had been completed, didn't seem phased by what I felt. I always tried to give as much information as I could when I was with medical specialists so that eventually something I said would spark a connection of some kind and enable them to put the pieces of my puzzle together to fix me. Most of the time, the specialists appeared neither interested nor able to do so. Once again, my mystery wasn't solved that day, but I was glad that the IV provided whatever my body had been lacking. At least this costly trip to the hospital had brought something good—something that so rarely happened for me after a visit to the doctor!

For the next few days, I considered everything that had taken place, searching for a reason why the IV would make such a difference. I'd been trying a Greens Diet during that time and had dramatically increased my intake of beet greens, bok choy, kale, and other greens. The naturopath I'd been working with over the phone had suggested that the only way for my body to heal was to flood it with nutrients. She believed that greens provide some of the best forms of healing energy—which I so desperately needed.

When I told her that I'd had difficulty tolerating these items in their raw states, she suggested that I steam them, then drink the juice that was created in the process instead.

It could be that these vegetables had upset a balance that the IV had restored. Whether that was true or not, I now had reservations about continuing to consume them in such great amounts. I wanted to continue the diet to provide my body with the nutrients needed to enable healing, but decided instead to adjust the amount and frequency of the greens, just in case. It wasn't long before another unusual symptom appeared. I began to wake at night with a relentless need to stretch my entire body. Within the week, I was waking several times a night for whole-body stretches. Soon, they were occurring not just during sleep but throughout the day as well.

One night during a stretching fit, I experienced an excruciating leg cramp. It seized my leg, but my whole body felt locked in its grip. The three minutes were an unbearable eternity. From that time on, before, during, and after any desire I had to stretch, the muscles throughout my whole body began to tighten, fearing another unbearable cramp. It was a tense existence, continually trying to relax my body while steeling myself against the possibility of incredible pain.

It was difficult enough avoiding "The Stretchies" when I was conscious, but it was really a challenge to try to control them while I was asleep. Some nights, I could sense them just lying in wait, like a cat crouched beside my bed, ready to pouch. No matter how much I felt the urge to stretch, I dared not move a muscle for fear that if I did, I would be overcome by another incredibly painful cramp.

When I told the naturopath about my unusual symptoms, she had never heard of such a response and was hesitant (though not in denial about the idea) that something so beneficial to most could be the cause of my problems. To us, though, the probability that the greens were involved seemed so high that we decided it would be best if I stopped taking them. So we gloomily thanked her for her time and efforts and resolved ourselves to the idea that we were back at square one.

Unfortunately, even though I discontinued the Green's Diet, The Stretchies, and their evil cousin, The Cramps, remained, although both were less intense and less frequent. In her quest for answers via the internet, Mary came across a health practitioner from Texas who believed that his unique prescription of Chinese medicine could restore my health. He offered a three-month protocol with a special blend of supplements. We both knew better than to think that I could handle medicine of any kind, but how would we know unless we tried? Once again, we were in the uncomfortable position of having to do something that wasn't likely to work just in case it did. In the past, it had always been frustrating and expensive—and our only option. This one took only a few days to explore because, almost immediately, my body made it clear that the medication wasn't a good fit. This guy and his ideas weren't going to work either.

Our next move was another naturopath, once again located in nearby Madison, Wisconsin. As we sat in the cramped and unassuming office while the receptionist finished the paperwork she'd been working on when we'd entered, we contemplated whether my chair wobbled because of the cracked floor beneath me or if one of the chair legs was shorter than the other. It was nice, actually, to come to places like this where the furniture and office space were simple and even somewhat defective because it showed that the people working there likely weren't in it for the money. Of course, I suppose one could consider that if they really knew what they were doing, they'd have more glamor. At this point, though, since we'd not experienced success with most of the specialists in so many of the fancy medical clinics we'd visited, it seemed good to be doing the opposite.

The receptionist eventually finished what she'd been working on and looked up at me. She introduced herself and began to ask me typical first-appointment questions, then handed me a shot-glass-sized cup and told me to spit in it until it was full. I was already intrigued and began to wonder if this might actually be a more scientific experience than the many appointments I had with western medical specialists.

When the cup was full, I gave it back to the receptionist. She informed me that after the saliva sample was analyzed, the results would be given to the naturopath, and she would meet with me to discuss them. It wasn't long before a woman appeared at the door and called my name. I followed her to another room where

I was asked to lay on a cot so she could take my blood pressure, which she explained would yield a more accurate result than one obtained while sitting.

Once she'd taken my vitals, the naturopath asked me what had brought me to her. She listened patiently as I told her about my history with Western Medicine. She was attentive and often nodded understandingly as I spoke of the many challenges I'd experienced. Her demeanor was a pleasant change from what I had experienced so many times during previous medical appointments. I never felt rushed, demeaned, or judged.

When I finished telling her about my condition, she began to explain the process she would be using to help me. The mainstay of her work, she said, involved live blood analysis. She would take a drop of blood from my finger, place it on a slide, then put it under a microscope. The image would then be projected onto her computer screen, which is where she would examine it and talk with me about what she had seen.

I'd always known about cells, of course, and the basics of how they look and what they do. These, however, weren't just any cells—they were my cells. My "right now" cells! Just seeing them was fascinating, but what she explained about the characteristics she noticed was even more captivating.

The naturopath told me that her job wasn't so much to diagnose a condition but rather to suggest supplements that would address the characteristics of the cells based on what she'd noticed from her examination of my blood and saliva. Although I'd had a lot of trouble with supplements in the past, she explained that these were selected specifically for me based on what she'd seen. In addition, each supplement was a single elemental nutrient rather than a synthetic composite, which should make it easier for my body to accept or, if there was trouble, to eliminate. She spoke confidently and enthusiastically. With all we'd seen and heard, it was easy to believe that we were on the right path, and we began to hope, once again, for a breakthrough.

The visit had been unusual and interesting but also quite expensive. Although our pocketbooks were light, our heads and hearts were full as we headed back to the car. I began to take the supplements right away. Apparently, her insight was correct because I was actually able to tolerate what she had suggested. I revisited her in the clinic for several months, and we repeated the same procedures. I always found the conversations interesting and her suggestions relevant. Each month, she would examine my blood cells in real-time and notice something new. It was absolutely fascinating. Unfortunately, after several months with no significant improvements, it seemed wise to stop, if only for a bit.

Once again, I began to feel overwhelmed. I wasn't just disappointed by this situation but by the fact that from a very short list of options, I now had one less. Faithfully, Mary didn't give up and continued her quest to leave no stone unturned as she hunted for new avenues of diagnosis and treatment. Along the way, we both couldn't shake our memory of the toxicology report I'd received nearly a year earlier. I recalled that before suggesting that we consult with a toxicologist, Doctor Aaron had initially suggested the help of Doctor M., a physician in a nearby community who worked in the area of integrative medicine. This meant that the doctor used a mixture of Eastern and Western approaches to healing. The testimonials on Doctor M's website were glowing. Many were from patients who claimed to have been sick and undiagnosed for years, and countless spoke of how Doctor M. had saved their lives. Mary called and got me in within the week. It seemed too good to be true, but I once again allowed myself to be cautiously optimistic.

Upon my arrival at Doctor M's practice, I read that his specialty was the treatment of Lyme disease. This was disappointing to me because I'd been tested for Lyme disease at least two times in the past and was assured that the results were negative each time. If something I didn't have was his focus, he might be unable to help me. I preferred a doctor with a wide base of knowledge. Still, if nothing else, he was licensed in western medicine, so the care would be covered by insurance, which was helpful. Who knows, I shrugged; maybe I would get lucky, and he would be the one. It was a desperate hope I'd had so many times before.

With this in mind, I was surprised and disappointed when I arrived for my appointment and was told that I would not actually be meeting Doctor M. but would instead be under the care of his assistant. Apparently, Doctor M. was a pretty hot commodity, so I would have to be satisfied to receive his expertise via his assistant. After expressing the concern that my complex situation would require the attention of an expert, the assistant assured me she would consult with Doctor M. along the way if needed but was confident that she had the necessary training to deal quite capably with things on her own.

My appointment went like many before it: a handful of forms, a ton of questions, my life history, and pinpointing events that seemed to be significant to my current health condition. I was sick, and sick of the same song and dance I had to go through at each new health practitioner we tried. When she wanted to give me a Lyme disease test, I told her I'd had these tests at least twice before, and both results showed I didn't have Lyme disease. Unfazed, she smiled and told me that this was a common response by her patients. She assured me that the Lyme disease test she would be giving me was far more accurate than the tests I had been given before. I didn't know there were different kinds of Lyme disease tests, so maybe this was a good sign. Of course, though, this one was more expensive than the others and wouldn't be covered by insurance.

I have endured a considerable amount of blood tests in my life and have been told more times than I can remember that just a few tests are required to check something or another. What it had always translated to in the past was a whole lot of money in exchange for little or no new relevant information. Needless to say, I wasn't thrilled about another high-priced test nor expecting to learn anything significant this time around. The doctor, however, was insistent—this test was crucial. She stressed the Lyme disease tests given by most physicians were inaccurate up to forty percent of the time and were especially erroneous if a person had been first infected with Lyme disease many years ago. My symptoms, she said, suggested that chronic Lyme disease could indeed be responsible for my lifelong health challenges, so there seemed to be no choice but to take the test. The assistant left, and a nurse returned who drew my blood. Before I left, I was asked to make an appointment to return in a month to hear the results and to begin treatment, if needed.

I returned a month later to discuss the result of the Lyme disease test. I was sure I was going to hear that the results were negative and that, according to my blood work, I was perfectly healthy. Or perhaps I'd find that the test results were inconclusive, but the clinic had an experimental therapy that could be just what I needed or a room full of supplements that could boost my system toward healing. In my mind, I was already projecting months into the future when I would be out a few thousand dollars—yet no healthier than I was now.

To my amazement, the assistant entered the room with a packet of papers and a confident smile. She told me she knew what was ailing me, that I had been suffering from *chronic* Lyme disease. Chronic Lyme disease, she said, often presents itself differently than Lyme disease discovered relatively quickly after the initial bite.

I cannot explain how elated I was! Finally, I knew what was wrong! This meant it could be properly treated. *Or could it? Could the doctor relieve the pain? When could we start? How long would it take?* My mind whirled with questions.

Unfortunately, the assistant's answers to my questions didn't provide the relief I was looking for. She explained that the initial symptoms of a bite vary; they generally cause fever, chills, severe headache, and achy joints, which can usually be eradicated. If, however, Lyme disease goes untreated for an extensive period of time, the situation becomes much more complex and is termed "chronic." Chronic Lyme disease is extremely difficult to eradicate because the bacteria becomes so deeply embedded into the system. The best course of treatment, I was told, was years of antibiotics, supplements, and other measures. Unfortunately, even with these protocols, some of my challenges would likely still remain.

After the initial thrill I'd felt about having the illness identified, news about its treatment came like a punch in the stomach. Even if I could afford the treatment, I'd likely have this condition for many more years to come and maybe even for the rest of my life. Even when the news about my health was good, it was still bad.

Chapter 18

The Disease That Never Was

For now we see in a mirror dimly, but then face to face; now I know in part, but then I will know fully, just as I also have been fully known.
1 Corinthians 13:12

On my next visit to Doctor M's clinic, I was told a blood test had confirmed there was another condition that could be contributing to my ill health. The test revealed I had hemochromatosis.

The disease, though difficult to pronounce, is apparently fairly easy to deal with—if you don't mind needles. Hemochromatosis is a blood disorder characterized by excess iron in the blood. Management of the disease simply required me to give a pint of blood every two weeks for twelve weeks, with a month break before the next twelve-week cycle. This blood-letting would drop my iron levels to normal, which was supposed to help with the chronic fatigue. It was important, I was told, to notify my siblings of the situation because since the condition was genetic, it was likely that one or more of them likely had it, too.

I made plans to begin the procedure right away but was told that I would need to wait about a week because the hospital in our small town did not stock the specific tubing and needles required. I didn't mind the wait, though, especially since it was easy for me to drive across town after work, have the blood drawn, and continue home rather than having to travel out of town to a larger city or facility to have it done. If all went well, my iron levels would stabilize after a few months, and I would need to go in less frequently. It was a little time-consuming, but the blood draws didn't bother me because it felt so good to be attacking the source of some of my health challenges. I anticipated the day my body began responding to the prescribed treatment, which would finally allow me some blessed relief from the "dis-ease" I had endured for so long. It almost seemed too good to be true.

Since the disease is hereditary, my doctor strongly encouraged me to notify my siblings of my condition and have them tested as well. Although I was really revved up to start getting after the chronic Lyme disease, Doctor M., via his assistant, insisted that it wouldn't be smart to begin the treatment until the hemochromatosis was under control, so that's what I did. After a month of blood draws, I returned to Doctor M's clinic for another consultation. Doctor M's assistant encouraged me to continue treating the hemochromatosis but was now willing also to treat the chronic Lyme disease. She prescribed the first antibiotic with the intention of adding a second in a few weeks and eventually another one until I was taking all three at once. This was a more cautious approach than I'd preferred (I just wanted to knock this thing out!), but she was the expert, so I went along with her plan.

In addition to her prescription for the first antibiotic, the assistant also suggested I begin a supplementation regime. Conveniently (for both of us, I think), there was an in-clinic pharmacy stocked floor to ceiling with bottles of all shapes, sizes, and purposes. By the number of supplements she'd prescribed, I knew I would be investing several hundred dollars, but what else could I do? I had to be all-in, or I might as well be out. As I handed my credit card to the clerk, I tried to block out the image of the unbelievable number of supplement bottles that already filled my kitchen cupboards at home.

When I got home, I removed all of the old supplements in a box and put them under my bed in case I might want to give one or more of them a try again later, then restocked the shelves with what I had brought home. I organized things so I'd be ready to start with the protocol the next morning. Upon awakening the next day, I carefully checked the instructions, doled out the many pills I'd need for breakfast and lunch, and went about my day. When I got home from work, I consulted the list again to figure out what I needed before, during, and after supper. I did the same the next day and the next.

At about this time, I became concerned with a small, painful area in my chest. It wasn't a new pain—I'd felt it frequently throughout the past twenty years or so. I'd been told it could be acid reflux, pneumonia, a hernia, or a buildup of cartilage near my breastbone, among other things. Even two emergency room visits with EKGs were inconclusive. This time, though, I was more worried about it than I'd been before because the pain was so intense and wouldn't go away.

Since typical first-line NSAIDs like ibuprofen, acetaminophen, and aspirin have always had a negative effect on my stomach, my head, or both—and often for me, didn't seem to have the pain-relief effect that I was seeking—I didn't even try any of them. I tried to deal with the discomfort by reassuring myself that it would eventually pass and by reminding myself that I'd been to the doctor so many times about the same thing in the past, and no one had been able to provide an effective treatment that I could tolerate on any of those visits, anyway. Still, I began to consider that maybe this time, the pain was a little different. Maybe it wasn't really the same thing I'd had in the past. Maybe it really was a warning sign for a serious heart condition. Over time, the excruciating pain and the worry that accompanied it grew even stronger. Mary scoured the internet for ideas, and I just tried to manage. We both prayed for strength, wisdom, and direction.

I was still certain a visit to a doctor who practiced Western medicine likely wouldn't help, but the pain was becoming unbearable so it was the easiest and quickest option. Maybe this time, it was the right choice for me. Very reluctantly, I agreed to have Mary schedule an appointment, which led to the next conundrum: Who should she call? The last clinic where the doctor indicated that my problems were all in my head or the one where the tests showed that my heart was in perfect condition? It wasn't a matter of insurance since Mary had pretty good coverage at that time, but rather a matter of my long and complicated medical history. I had seen almost every doctor in the community at least once, and they all seemed to think I was making everything up, so Mary and I knew we had to be strategic.

We finally settled on the idea of visiting a newly-constructed clinic in our hometown. We hoped that the doctors would be new to the area and, therefore, wouldn't have access to my extensive medical records, which I thought might contain information that hinted that my physical health was related more to my mental health than anything else.

Mary wasn't able to go with me to my appointment, so I was on my own that day, and I felt a little alone as I walked down the hall to the receptionist. It was not very busy at that time of the day, so it wasn't long before a nurse called my name, and I found myself seated in the inner waiting room with a nurse who was taking my vitals. All, of course, were within the normal range, which always seemed to frustrate me because I most certainly didn't feel "normal."

The physician was just closing my file as he entered the room. Apparently, he'd gotten information from an affiliate clinic in a different location because, being that it was my first visit there, there shouldn't have been much for him to peruse. He'd barely put eyes on me and didn't even offer a greeting before brusquely asking, "So, what is it you think you have?" I was taken aback by his manner but tried not to let the coldness of his tone irritate me as I began to describe the lingering chest discomfort that had brought me there, along with other information that seemed relevant to the situation. I had learned by then to be careful with my words so that I revealed just enough to be helpful without going so far into my history to sound looney.

The sneer the doctor seemed to enter the room with only seemed to grow as I explained about my recent diagnosis of hemochromatosis and chronic Lyme disease. When he heard me mention these prognoses, the doctor reopened the file folder as if looking for more information about each condition.

"Who diagnosed you with this?" he barked.

When I explained where I'd learned about the conditions, the physician shook his head with a smirk. "Well, first of all," he almost chuckled, "you don't have hemochromatosis." He opened the file folder once again and pointed at my blood test results on the paperwork inside, highlighting that the data needed to prove its presence simply was not there. He barely paused before going on to launch another verbal shot my way.

"So, I'm going to take a wild guess and say the same clinic also diagnosed you with chronic Lyme disease?"

I nodded, my sinking stomach almost overriding my irritation at the man. "Well," he continued, "ever since Doctor M. opened his clinic, everybody seems to have chronic Lyme disease." He looked at me squarely, "But you don't have that, either." He must have been having a great time with the situation because he couldn't seem to contain his mirth. For the next minute or so, he continued to belittle the idea of chronic Lyme disease, emphasizing that it was just a fallacy—a diagnosis thrown at people without merit. "It's just not true," he grinned one last time as if banging the final nail in the coffin.

I could hardly believe my ears. It's one thing to leave a doctor's office without a doctor being able to determine what was causing discomfort or being able to alleviate an illness—something I'd done many, many times. It was quite another thing, though, to feel outright criticized and ridiculed there.

When I got home, I called Mary right away. By then, any irritation I'd felt at the clinic had already turned to utter sadness. Mary, however, was irate! She couldn't believe the doctor just told me I didn't have either condition—and had done it so callously. It was one thing for him not to know much about chronic Lyme disease or even to doubt its existence, as so many others at that time were doing. Nonetheless, how could he deny the diagnosis of hemochromatosis? What did he mean by stating that the markers on my blood test actually denied its presence?

At this point, it was clear a reasonable next step would be clarification from Doctor M's clinic. Since it was too late to contact them that day, Mary told me she'd do so right when it opened the next morning. We were confident they'd be able to set that doctor, and his bad attitude, straight.

At 8:00 a.m. the next morning, Mary placed the call. She stated what had occurred with the doctor at my appointment the previous day and said she wanted to talk to the doctor or a nurse about it as soon as possible. The receptionist transferred the call to the nurse, who relayed the information a second time. The nurse asked Mary to wait just a moment for her to peruse the information, then asked for her patience once again while she consulted a second nurse.

After several minutes, someone else took over the conversation. This person matter-of-factly stated that the doctor I'd seen the previous day was right: I didn't actually *have* hemochromatosis, but I did have *one* of the markers for it.

Mary could hardly believe her ears. What did this person mean that I didn't actually *have* hemochromatosis? Why had we been told that I did, and more importantly, why had we paid to have blood drawn for weeks and weeks as treatment for the disease if I didn't have it? Why had I been asked to delay treatment of the chronic Lyme disease until it could be brought under control? Why had I been told to contact all seven of my siblings so they could be tested for it, too, if it wasn't something that actually existed in my body?

When Mary called me to share what she had learned, I was incredulous. I believed her, of course, but there had to be some kind of misunderstanding or something missing in the explanation that I needed to hear. If there wasn't, I needed to hear that, too. So I called the clinic myself only to hear what seemed to be the exact same information.

While the nurse talked, I couldn't help but think of the embarrassing phone calls I would soon need to make to each of my siblings, apologizing for advising them to spend time and money on tests for a condition they weren't likely to have—while considering all the time and money I'd spent myself. Most of all, though, I was becoming extremely agitated that the medical personnel at the clinic had been either wrong or dishonest about my condition. At that moment, it didn't seem to matter if the medical staff had been incompetent or dishonest. What did matter was that my hope for healing had all but evaporated.

During the nurse's attempt to explain the misinformation, it became clear to me what the truth had been and that I was again being manipulated. I became furious. I raised my voice and struggled to control my emotions. I struggled to control what I said and how I said it. "I feel like suing the clinic for what you've put me through!" I said, venting my frustration loudly.

I had barely finished my sentence before the nurse quickly interrupted me to announce that because I'd used the word "sue," our conversation was done, and she hung up the phone. I could hardly believe what had just occurred—from the information I'd received to the conversation's abrupt ending. I could only stand, shocked, with the phone to my ear for several more moments in disbelief.

The next day, I was surprised to receive a phone call from Doctor M's clinic. I was told in no uncertain terms that the word "sue" was not tolerated, and once it was uttered by a client, all ties with that individual would immediately be severed. By this time, I'd begun to feel some remorse about how I'd handled myself during that phone call. I guess there were two reasons for this. First, I wasn't happy that I'd used such a harsh tone, and second, I realized that I was now unable to proceed in their care for chronic Lyme disease, which was their specialty. I found some comfort in the fact that the comprehensive nature of their reply indicated that I wasn't likely the first to have interacted with them in this way. Still, this comfort was overshadowed by the grim realization that the only practitioner who recognized my illness as a valid disease was no longer available to help me. I sank back into the chair and dropped my face into my hands. *What was I going to do?* My diagnosis and treatment plan at Doctor M's practice had offered a glimmer of hope which was now completely extinguished. Healing—and God—seemed a million miles away.

Chapter 19

Into the Storm

My heart is in anguish within me, and the terrors of death have fallen upon me. Fear and trembling come upon me, and horror has overwhelmed me. I said, "Oh, that I had wings like a dove! I would fly away and be at rest. Behold, I would flee far away, I would spend my nights in the wilderness. I would hurry to my place of refuge from the stormy wind and heavy gale.
Psalm 55:4-8

One would think that after floundering in despair so many times before, I would have realized God was always with me and would never abandon me. I was so exhausted, however, from the ever-present battles I faced that my endurance was limited and my hope almost nonexistent. Thankfully Mary still had some hope in reserve because she immediately began to search for alternatives. We were both surprised, in fact, when she rather quickly discovered that there was another physician not so far away who'd earned acclaim for his treatment of chronic Lyme disease. His name was Doctor John Hoffman, and his clinic was in Waupaca—only an hour from our home.

As quickly as our hopes had risen with this news, however, they were immediately dashed when a closer examination of the clinic's website indicated that his caseload was full and he was not taking on any new patients. Regardless, with fingers crossed, Mary dialed the clinic early the next day to see if she could convince the receptionist to squeeze in just one more sick being. Imagine her surprise when none other than the doctor himself answered. He listened intently as Mary briefly explained my health history and current plight. His response? "Come into the clinic next week to begin treatment." When she relayed the news to me, I could hardly believe my ears. I wouldn't even have been able to get into Doctor M's clinic that quickly, even if they'd still allowed me there.

Although I would have been thrilled if I could have gone directly to the appointment that same day, having a little time to prepare was good because I needed to arrange for my files to be sent from Doctor M's clinic and from any other physicians that seemed relevant. Mary also suggested that I keep a food journal for a few days in hopes that Doctor Hoffmann could use the information there to help me diversify my diet. So we spent the week gathering the information we needed along with making a list of questions we had about my situation that we hoped to ask during our time with the doctor.

On Monday morning, we left at sunrise to be sure we wouldn't be late for our appointment in the unfamiliar town. We arrived before the clinic opened and waited excitedly but cautiously in the car as the minutes ticked slowly toward 8:00 a.m. Eventually, we noticed a woman unlocking the main door, so we exited the car and entered the building.

The clinic consisted of a few small rooms in what likely had once been someone's home. Doctor Hoffman shared the space with another business on the other side of the building, which we noticed as we followed a rather twisted path through the short, narrow hallways and down a small set of stairs. The receptionist behind the counter welcomed us and invited us to take a seat on one of the well-worn yet functional chairs in the waiting room a few feet away until the doctor was ready to meet with us.

Doctor Hoffman was a quiet, unassuming older man with snowy hair contrasting a sun-weathered face. He walked with the speed and posture of someone who had just dismounted a horse after a long day on the trail. When he approached us, he was accompanied by a pleasant middle-aged woman dressed in blue jeans, a long-sleeved shirt, and a quilted vest. He introduced himself briefly but then left to attend to another couple who had arrived shortly after we'd been seated. The middle-aged woman then smiled warmly and invited us to follow her to a tiny room a few steps away.

Once we were settled in our places, the woman introduced herself. She explained that she was a nurse practitioner working under the guidance of Doctor Hoffmann. She told us she'd begun to study chronic Lyme disease after her daughter had been diagnosed with the condition several years earlier. By this time, she'd studied the disease extensively, including having traveled to learn from some of the leading specialists in the country. As a result, she not only had a wealth of knowledge but a passion to provide desperately-needed treatment for those suffering from the terrible condition. By this time, Mary and I could already see and feel her kindness and intelligence and knew we were in good hands.

Rebecca, our nurse, lived about five hours away in northern Wisconsin but traveled to Waupaca for a few days every month to learn from Doctor Hoffmann. In doing so, she was able to help him manage his growing caseload. She was well aware of the complications of chronic Lyme disease—especially its unusual and widely-varying symptoms. She also knew about the lack of response and disrespect most physicians show to those who suffer from it. More importantly, Rebecca knew how extremely difficult it was to return someone afflicted with the disease to good health. While I was thrilled to find such an expert, the more I learned, the more I realized the tough road ahead of me.

Doctor M. and the other clinics from which I'd requested my files had sent them ahead of me. Since my blood work was quite recent, neither Doctor Hoffman nor Rebecca thought it was necessary for me to do anymore. *Another good sign,* Mary and I agreed with a glance. We know that most places would have ordered new tests whether I needed them or not. Rebecca then opened my file folder and showed me how the different bands of color in the test results confirmed a positive Lyme disease diagnosis several times over. She explained the results indicated my tick bite had likely occurred many years ago, perhaps even as far back as early childhood, which was one reason why mainstream tests had shown a false negative. In addition, my condition was complicated by the fact that I was also likely suffering from one or more co-infections caused by bacteria that had entered my body from the very same tick bite (or perhaps even from a second tick bite). These co-infections were causing other diseases, such as Babesia and Bartonella, which could be as debilitating as the chronic Lyme disease itself, if not even more challenging to eradicate.

Perhaps the most refreshing part of this clinic experience was that at no time during the appointment did I feel my time was limited or that Rebecca was in a hurry. Not once did I get the impression my questions were stupid or that my complaints were invalid. In fact, Rebecca focused solely on Mary and me in every moment, spoke empathetically, and exhibited encyclopedic knowledge about chronic Lyme disease. She was not only smart and experienced—she was also compassionate and creative. She looked me in the eye and listened to me talk about my symptoms as no one had for years. I could not remember when I'd last had care like that.

After about an hour with Rebecca, we sensed she was finishing her time with us, so we began to gather our things. Just then, however, Doctor Hoffman walked through the door, meandered toward us, and took a seat. Rebecca briefed him about what we'd discussed and shared her plan of action with him. Doctor Hoffman took a few moments to consider her plan in light of my particular test results and soon nodded in agreement. He confirmed everything Doctor M. and Rebecca had said but added two things I hadn't heard before. "First," he explained, "it's important for you to know that healing a body from chronic Lyme disease is like peeling an onion. There are lots and lots of layers, and as a result, it takes a long time to eradicate it." I nodded and grimaced at the same time. He continued as if to punctuate the challenge ahead of me. "There is nothing you can do but peel the layers away one at a time." He looked me in the eye until he was sure I understood. "Second," he continued, "your condition is going to get *worse* before it gets better." He again paused to let that sink in. "This is because the treatment involves killing the Lyme bacteria. When they die, they release a toxic waste product. This condition is referred to as the Herxheimer reaction, and it is no laughing matter." He could see in my face I was paying close attention and that I was already somewhat troubled by the news, then went on. "In the coming weeks, you likely will not be able to tell if you're feeling lousy because you're getting better or feeling lousy because you're getting worse. It will only be in time that we will really know."

"So what am I to do?" I asked, much like a child to a parent, seeking not just advice but reassurance

"Just proceed as if you're headed in the right direction, no matter how uncomfortable you get," the doctor replied. "If the pain eventually subsides, the treatment is gaining success. If not. . ." he shrugged with a frown that said, "We can only try."

Mary squeezed my hand, and I took a deep breath. As bad as it sounded, I knew there was no other direction to go but forward—straight into the storm. I consented to treatment, and Doctor Hoffmann wrote me a prescription for three different antibiotics. He then told me to persevere, shook my hand, and sent me on my way.

Before leaving the clinic, I made an appointment to revisit the clinic in a month. As Mary and I headed back to our car, it was hard not to recognize the gravity of this moment. While it was undoubtedly a routine day for Doctor Hoffmann and Rebecca, it was a huge one for me. Finally, I felt as if I was taking a step forward on a path that so often went sideways or backward for me. Just maybe this would finally be the beginning of the end of my suffering—a concept that seemed almost too good to be true.

It took me a while to gather the courage needed to begin taking the antibiotics Doctor Hoffman had prescribed. I was just too fearful of the "getting worse before getting better" part to begin. Honestly, I wasn't even sure my body could handle much "worse" than what it was already going through. Eventually, though, I knew I had to give it a try, so as prescribed, I took the first antibiotic. Then, after a week, I took the second. Then I waited another week and began the third.

To my surprise, the first few weeks weren't so bad. I actually felt pretty good compared to how I usually felt. I didn't know it then, but this was a honeymoon period of sorts because although the antibiotics were steadily attacking the Lyme disease bacteria in my cells, the amount of waste product hadn't yet accumulated to a level that was great enough to cause a noticeable Herxheimer reaction. In addition, just as Rebecca had predicted, some of the bacteria had been able to hide from the antibiotic in order to remain unaffected by it. I could almost picture those nasty little critters huddled together in some safe location inside my body, laughing at how they'd outsmarted the medicine I'd been taking to destroy them and plotting about how they would take revenge upon it—upon me.

By week three, it was obvious that I'd killed enough bacteria to reach the threshold of Herxheimer discomfort, and the rest of the bacteria—the ones who'd initially gone into hiding—appeared now to be angry. Very angry. Because this resulted in considerable suffering for me, it made me angry, too. More than anger, however, it brought sadness and reaffirmed past desires for my own death because it was the only thing that seemed to offer relief. During this period, every symptom I'd ever experienced returned, but this time each one was at least twice as bad as it had originally felt. My brain was foggy, and I was continually nauseous and achy. I was exhausted, but I couldn't sleep. I was hungry, but my body seemed to have a negative response to almost everything I ate. I could hardly face the thought of having to endure this level of discomfort for years on end, slowly peeling and peeling away those onion layers until *maybe* someday I'd eventually get at least a little better. Unless, of course, the dangerous effect of taking too many antibiotics for too long didn't do me in somehow before that.

Perhaps the only thing going for me at this point was the fact that I'd been sad for so long that my current level of despondency couldn't get much lower. What I didn't know, however, was where my current level of physical discomfort fell in relation to where it could potentially be. Nor how much joint pain, chest pain, head pain, muscle pain, stomach pain, back pain, nerve pain, or eye pain I could handle. Further, what if all of these pains one day decided to all descend upon me at the exact same moment?

I didn't have to wonder long about my personal pain tolerance level or the ultimate level of pain ahead of me because one morning, I woke up to pure, unadulterated agony coursing through my entire body. It was everywhere, and it was almost unbearable.

Between groaning, crying, and writhing in pain, I increasingly began to flop out of bed, fall on my knees, and plead with God. I begged Him to either take me or heal me. I had prayed daily for years, but as this storm intensified, so did my prayers. In the midst of my cries for help, however, I recognized a feeling of complete and utter loneliness. *Where was God?* my mind demanded. *Why had He left me so alone when I needed Him so desperately?* In addition to chastising Him, I considered how exasperated I felt toward the humans in my life who also weren't providing me with the level of comfort and compassion I desired. I looked at Mary lying right beside me and wondered critically if she was praying for me as intently and as often as she should be. My thoughts then moved to my parents: *Did they even care about my misery? How about my siblings, my friends, and my co-workers?* All of them seemed to be going on with their lives as if I wasn't experiencing mental and physical pain that was almost unbearable. It seemed that I'd been left to live this tortuous existence all by myself, and I felt so desperately alone.

Every day, after a few minutes of contemplation and prayer, there wasn't much else for me to do but struggle to my feet, put on as happy a face as possible, and head out into the day—agony and all. When I was greeted with the standard "How are you doing?" I'd learned to pretend everything was fine because, quite frankly, it gets old explaining the details of what I was facing to someone, then the next, over and over again. In addition, it had quickly become evident that *few* people really wanted to know how I was doing. At first, when asked, I'd answer truthfully and begin to explain in full my mental and physical condition. I was thankful that I could talk about my situation and relieved, somehow, that in telling it to others, I could unload some of my burden. Most responded with a few comforting or encouraging words. In the end, however, the majority of those I talked with indicated that they had neither the time nor the interest in hearing the real story of what I was experiencing, so I learned to just try to smile and keep things brief instead.

I don't know if the second antibiotic was worse than the first, but before long, I could no longer tolerate the level of pain I was experiencing. I couldn't concentrate on anything because I was suffering so much. When the pain of one side effect became so brutal, I broke down into tears, and I knew I couldn't continue. I decided to stop taking the third antibiotic to see if that might alleviate some of my symptoms. Of course, I worried that I might be prolonging my healing, but there didn't seem to be any alternative. I hoped I'd be feeling well enough within a week to try again, although honestly, the thought of that was overwhelming.

In reality, I didn't even begin taking the third antibiotic again before it was time for my second appointment with Rebecca and Doctor Hoffman, and I was a little nervous to tell them because I wasn't sure how they'd take the news that I'd stopped. Based on what I'd learned about them at the first appointment, I should have known better than to expect criticism or irritation from them about this or any other choice I made regarding my treatment. Rebecca and the good doctor were always on my side. They always listened intently and made decisions for me based on my symptoms and current tolerance level. Two things were quickly obvious with them. First, they really did want to relieve the dis-ease that I felt. They weren't in this for the money or the fame or anything else. Second, there was no standard plan for getting through this illness. They highlighted this once again at this second appointment. The healing process was different from person to person.

To my tremendous relief, Rebecca and Doctor Hoffman told me I didn't have to restart taking the third antibiotic—not now, anyway. They encouraged me instead to continue taking the two antibiotics for now. In the future, we could add the third— or maybe something else. As we left the clinic for the second time, Mary and I knew we were fortunate to have found these experts. Doctor Hoffmann and Rebecca had so much insight and experience about chronic Lyme disease, but more than anything else, they truly cared.

After a few months of intensive treatment of the chronic Lyme disease itself, Rebecca and Doctor Hoffmann began to address some of the possible co-infections that were plaguing me. My symptoms suggested Babesia and Bartonella. Babesia bacteria are related to the bacteria responsible for malaria. Both are characterized by drenching sweats, pain around the heart, headaches, muscle aches, and fatigue. On the other hand, symptoms of Bartonella include streaked rashes, lower abdominal pain, sore soles, tender lymph nodes in the extremities, a sore throat, and, once again, fatigue. If there was a Lyme disease lottery, I had apparently won the mega-jackpot—I had all three co-infections and possibly others. Strangely, this news was somewhat comforting as at least we knew what was afflicting me. It made sense that symptoms kept changing due to the co-infections. Of course, all of this made my climb toward healing seem even steeper, yet I knew that there was only one way to good health, and that was straight up. So once again, I steeled myself for a tough battle and proceeded ahead.

Over the next year, I continued working with Doctor Hoffman and Rebecca whenever she was in town during my appointment. If the pain or discomfort became too much, the dose or frequency were adjusted. As I continued treatment, it became apparent I was far from alone in my struggle against chronic Lyme disease. Every time I visited the clinic, I saw or heard of others who had been dealing with the same struggles. I was humbled to notice that some appeared to be suffering far worse than me, at least outwardly anyway. A few were partially or totally paralyzed, while others showed signs of significant mental impairment. Most of the time, though, it was intriguing how healthy many of the patients all appeared from the outside. In fact, Mary and I often made guesses about which one was the sick one and which one was accompanying the patient when pairs arrived at an appointment. "Was it him or his wife?" Astonishingly, we were wrong more often than we were right.

Perhaps because I was immersed in treatment for chronic Lyme disease during this time, Mary and I began to hear more and more about the condition on the news, and much to our surprise, many of the patients' stories closely mirrored my own. While it was comforting to hear of so many others who shared my experience, it made me angry to think about how many of them (of us) had been told that there was nothing wrong with them despite their near-constant misery. Added to my contempt was frustration with those who seemed so quick to designate me as having mental issues rather than physical ones and how much money all of us had spent in our futile search for relief. The bright side, of course, was that at least some of that was behind us now. Mary and I knew we'd been extremely blessed to find the terrific care I was now receiving from Rebecca and Doctor Hoffmann.

Although it was the knowledge of Doctor Hoffmann that had brought me to the clinic, I began to work more and more exclusively with Rebecca over time. This was fine with us because she was exceptionally insightful, attentive, and kind, and we genuinely admired her. She was still under Doctor Hoffman's watch for legal purposes and probably consulted with him regularly about all of us, but eventually she began to consult and prescribe protocols with increasing independence. Soon, Rebecca herself became a highly sought-after resource in Wisconsin, which seemed to fuel an even greater desire in her to help those who were suffering. Her home and clinic were in the far northern reaches of the state, so she decided to set up an office in Pewaukee for one week every other month. She'd drive down to the city the Sunday before and stay in a hotel throughout the week of appointments there. Occasionally she'd return to Waupaca to help Doctor Hoffmann, but for the most part, she was now on her own in these two locations.

An appointment at her clinic in Pewaukee was more convenient for me than it would have been if I'd had to travel to the far northern reaches of the state, but it likely wasn't the most convenient situation for Rebecca. I always marveled that she never showed even an ounce of irritation over the disruption it likely brought to her life. To Mary and me, Rebecca was the embodiment of what it meant to care for the sick. She may not have been a physician by legal standards, but she was more of a doctor than most I'd ever visited.

By the time I was making monthly visits to see Rebecca in Pewaukee, I'd managed to start a consistent routine of taking three or four antibiotics at a time. Despite so much that was good about my treatment, my path toward healing was still far from smooth. I was physically making only small improvements, which were often followed by a similar-sized setback in one way or another. Overall, though, I no longer felt as if each new day might be my last, which was a big plus for me, and over time, it was clear that I'd actually made significant progress. Remarkably, the benefits weren't just physical. I actually started looking forward to some things I'd previously been too tired—or in too much pain—to appreciate: golfing with my friends, playing catch with the boys, and taking Sunday drives through the countryside with Mary. At work, I was laughing more and was a little less irritable toward my co-workers. Somewhere along the way, I even began to entertain hopes and dreams again. It's a good thing I was feeling this way because Mary was developing some incredible hopes and dreams of her own

Chapter 20

Desires of the Heart

*Pure and undefiled religion in the sight
of our God and Father is this: to visit
orphans and widows in their distress, and
to keep oneself unstained by the world.*
James 1:27

For many years, Mary carried a list of desires in her heart. I was aware of most of them, but there were some that she hadn't yet shared with me or anyone else. I knew she wanted to travel, renovate the house, and one day, perhaps, even relocate to the country. Unfortunately, my health—or lack of it—came with an incredibly high price tag, so Mary had been forced to put most of her dreams on hold for a long time. Even if we'd had the money (which we didn't because so much of it was spent on trying to get me well), significant travel required so much planning and uncertainty that it sucked most of the fun out of it for me anyway. Also, my diet was so restricted there was no way I could get what I needed from a restaurant or anywhere else on the go. Likewise, when any one or more of my symptoms randomly appeared, which they typically seemed to do, it would definitely be uncomfortable to be driving, sightseeing, or anywhere except for my bed. As disappointing as it was, it just seemed easier to stay home.

Of course, this didn't deter Mary. While at home, she often dreamed of exotic places we would go to if we had all the time, money, and health in the world. It wasn't just the international locations she was pining for; she longed to meet the people, eat the food, and see the everyday sights in other parts of the world. She was especially drawn to the children in other locales. First, she read a book about a woman who'd opened her home to orphaned African children. Then she found the website of a woman who'd traveled to Uganda as a missionary and then adopted one, two, three . . . thirteen children, all while she was not yet even thirty years old. Somewhere along the way and unbeknownst to me, Mary began to explore African orphanages. Some of the orphanages had photo listings of the children in their care. In every little face, Mary saw the heart and soul of a beautiful child of God.

Mary began casually showing me pictures and bringing up cute anecdotes written about the children while I was watching TV or making supper. I guess I was still clueless, and when I didn't get the hint, Mary overtly suggested how one or the other might fit in perfectly with our family. Eventually, I got it, and my response was blunt, "We don't have enough money for that right now, and I'm just not healthy enough, anyway." I suggested that in a few years—if I felt better—we could begin talking seriously about adopting one of those children. I surely wasn't very sensitive about how disappointing this must have been for Mary. Nonetheless, she wasn't one to give up that easily, and just as she'd stuck with me for better and worse through my illness, she kept on with her dream: reading, researching, and looking at photos.

In August 2010, Mary called me over as she brought up some information on her laptop. "John! You have to come and take a look at this cutie," she said. *Oh boy,* I thought. *Here we go again.* As I trudged over, I had already begun to load my response, but before I said anything, I looked over her shoulder and peered at the screen. On it, I saw a boy about nine or ten years old. My intended response—the words I had spoken many times before—didn't make their way out of my mouth. Instead, as I looked a little longer and more closely, something strange happened in my heart—something almost miraculous. As I looked at this little boy's smiling face, all of my problems faded into the background, replaced by a disarming sense of joy. His little face was just so sweet and innocent despite the trying conditions he'd likely experienced in his young lifetime.

Almost without thinking, I heard myself say the words I never thought would come out of my mouth, "Mary, I think we should do it! We should adopt him."

I'm not sure who was more surprised at my response. In hindsight, the moment actually seems a little surreal. I remember saying the words, looking at Mary, and being totally at peace with the thought. It wasn't scary, overwhelming, or worrisome. In those few moments, neither my health nor the legal cost of the process came anywhere near our minds. I can only conclude that's how it goes when you follow God's plan for your life. You just yield to it and let Him carry you along the path He would have you take. I was simply listening to God, and my wife was looking at me like some sort of knight in shining armor.

When I looked at the boy in the picture, two things happened: first, I instantly knew he was my son; second, any doubts about being too sick or lacking the necessary funds were overshadowed by the thought *that this is a situation that is so much bigger than me. It's from God, and everything about it will be okay if we just trust Him.* God sure does make His plan plain and clear sometimes.

The boy was from an orphanage in the small town of Yako in the country of Burkina Faso in West Africa. Neither Mary nor I had even heard of Burkina Faso and had no idea where it was in Africa. Suddenly my mind began to take over. Although I hadn't felt even the least bit of concern when I told Mary this was a good idea for us, doubt started creeping into my mind. I began to be concerned about my health and my ability to take on such a tremendous challenge while dealing with such significant other challenges every day. I also couldn't help but wonder if our family was stable enough to handle the disruption of the new addition and, most of all, if we could afford it. I had many concerns, and my mind began to reel. As it did, though, I thought back to the moment I first saw his face, and I simply knew it was the will of God. As nerve-wracking as it was, I chose to focus on that instead of my worries.

Ferdinand had lived at the orphanage in Yako for several years. Since we knew very little about him, we had many questions. Some were large, with answers that had the potential to stop or at least give us cause to slow down and reconsider: *Has Ferdinand ever been physically abused? Does he respect authority? Will he, after all he has been through, be able to attach and assimilate into a new family? How traumatized is he, and how has this affected him?* Others were smaller in significance but intriguing because of what they would reveal about him: *How tall is he? What is his favorite food? What does his laugh sound like? Is he kind? Is he timid or macho? What sports does he enjoy?*

Our contact in Burkina Faso was the original founder of the orphanage, school, and clinic, a wonderfully dedicated woman named Ruth. Mary and I sent Ruth email after email, trying our best to keep our questions to those only of necessity so as not to overwhelm her. Ruth responded readily to every message as if we were her number one priority. We later discovered how many other people she was conversing with and the numerous other responsibilities she had. I had not seen someone who truly exemplified God's love so deeply in a long, long time.

Over the next few weeks, Mary and I were more and more convinced that we would eventually proceed with the adoption, but we hadn't formally committed to it yet because we wanted to be sure we could financially and emotionally provide for his needs. It was easy to start to give in to nagging thoughts and fears about the situation and why this may not be right for us: *Would this be detrimental to our family unit? Would it be good for Ferdie? What challenges would be faced raising a black son in an overwhelmingly white population?*

Occasionally, we'd email Ruth to ask her thoughts about one concern or another. She was always so gracious and forthcoming with her responses from Ferdie's point of view, and said adoption was absolutely the right choice. In Africa, she said, even orphans who are fortunate enough to be cared for in an orphanage during childhood face extreme difficulty when they become adults because they ultimately must venture out and face the world on their own. Unlike peers who live with their families, orphans don't have the opportunity to work their father's plot of land or to help in the family business, so they must take jobs at the lowest end of society, working as street vendors or domestic servants or in unregulated and dangerous trades such as mining or commercial farming. Of course, many young adult orphans would eventually find themselves in the worst-case scenario: in the world of drugs or sex trafficking. Ruth's reassurance reinforced the message I'd heard in my mind the first time I saw the boy's photo (and was reminded of frequently afterward): *This is a situation that is so much bigger than me. It's from God, and everything about it will be okay if we just trust Him.*

After much prayer and discussion, on Christmas Day 2010, Mary contacted Ruth and joyfully told her we wanted to adopt Ferdinand, the smiling boy in the photo Mary had shown me many weeks earlier. Mary often says that from the time the "yes" was given, it was as if the rug was pulled out from under us, and we were swept away on the journey forward to reaching our new son. I think it began way before that, though, with our first glimpse of Ferdie, the one where I immediately recognized that I was looking into my son's eyes.

The adoption process moved quickly, although, for all the busy work involved, the truth remained that there was much time and considerable luck standing between our family and Ferdie. Mary aggressively filled out paperwork, got documents notarized, sent money, and made appointments at government offices to meet the process's many requirements. It was confusing and overwhelming every step of the way. Almost every piece of paperwork seemed to require some amount of guesswork regarding exactly what was expected. All we could do was send a good deal of prayer along with the documents each time in hopes that the papers wouldn't be returned to us to be completed again due to one error or another.

My emotions fluctuated over the next few months. I sometimes felt positive about our plans, but at other times, I admit I felt pretty anxious. *How are we going to afford the adoption? Am I healthy enough emotionally and physically to support another child? Is my body strong enough to tolerate the immunizations needed to travel to Burkina Faso? If so, would my immune system be able to manage the "bugs" in a new and very different land, and what will I eat when I am there?* These thoughts bounced back and forth depending on how I felt. That is, how I felt—not God. His thoughts and words remained constant, each time, in one way or another: *This is a situation that is so much bigger than me, but it's from God, and everything about it will be okay if we just trust Him.* Still, I was about to face some health complications that would make me wonder if someone was playing a huge joke on me.

Chapter 21

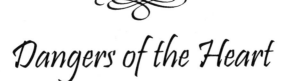

Dangers of the Heart

These things I have spoken to you so that in Me you may have peace. In the world you have tribulation, but take courage; I have overcome the world.
John 16:33

Despite the confidence I had that the adoption was the right thing to do, I was still often concerned about how my health challenges would impact the situation. Although I'd found the main cause of and a great solution to my problem, my improvements started to slow. It was soon clear that I'd reached a plateau yet was far from healed. I also noticed that my body had an interesting reaction to the antibiotics. At first, each one would be effective, yet once I stopped taking the antibiotic to begin a new one that would attack a different symptom, I would again experience the symptoms I'd had in the first place. It was as if the bacteria had just gone into hiding for a while until the coast was clear, then returned in full force as it was rather than being fully eradicated.

I also had trouble tolerating the dosages prescribed for me. Symptoms included trouble urinating, inflamed and painful lower legs, stiff joints, and continual digestive distress. I presented my concerns to Rebecca at my next appointment, who suggested a new plan of attack. She proposed inserting a PICC (peripherally inserted central catheter) line through the vein in my arm. The antibiotics would then be administered through the line and directly into my bloodstream, thereby no longer requiring me to swallow the antibiotic pills. This would bypass my digestive system where the medication seemed to be causing so much distress. Her solution sounded almost too good to be true.

Rebecca sent me on the way with a detailed explanation of my next steps for the PICC line treatment. I had to find a surgeon to insert the line, and place an order with a distributor that would sell the liquid antibiotics to me. I also had to schedule in-home nurse visits to advise me how to inject the medication, keep the area clean, and change the bandaging. Then I had to call to my insurance company to explain the situation and make sure it would be covered. It was a rather overwhelming to-do list because there were so many unknowns. In many cases, I wasn't really sure what I was asking for and of whom I was supposed to be asking it.

We started by finding a local surgeon who was willing to perform the procedure. At that time, a PICC line—especially one inserted for the purpose of antibiotic treatment of chronic Lyme disease—was not only unusual but also rather controversial because, once again, many doctors simply didn't believe that chronic Lyme disease was a real condition. Luckily for us, we were able to find someone right at our local hospital who was able (and willing) to insert the line within just a few weeks' time.

On the day of the procedure, I made the short five-block drive to the hospital and checked myself in. I was eventually shown to the pre-op room, where I was given a gown and a bed and asked to wait for further instructions. When it was my turn, I was wheeled to the operating room and given local anesthesia a few minutes before the surgeon began to insert the line. The procedure was amazingly quick. Almost before I knew it, the PICC line had been inserted into a vein in my left arm, then pushed through to the large central veins near my heart. I was then wheeled back to the recovery room where I rested briefly and waited for a nurse to confirm that all was well. Before being released, I was given a quick demonstration of how to administer the daily intravenous antibiotics and how to change the dressing, which would have to be done every third day to prevent infection.

The learning curve involved in living with a PICC line was steep. Cleaning the site and changing the bandaging without pulling out the line was tricky, as was showering without getting it wet, not to mention walking around with short sleeves without it being a topic of conversation wherever I went. My first independent antibiotic injections were tentative and clumsy, but I did the best I could and felt that, overall, I was able to do what I recall being shown. I got a little better at it with each subsequent injection and pretty soon felt I was getting into a routine. Nothing about the PICC line was easy or comfortable, but it was what I needed to do and I was hopeful that it would eventually lead me to better health.

For the next few weeks, I muddled along as well as I could. I was pleased to have a treatment option that bypassed my stomach so my body was better able to tolerate the prescribed dosages, and I continually reminded myself how fortunate I was to have this option. The truth was, though, that the line was irritating and cumbersome, as was the elastic sleeve I wore to cover it from public view. In addition, every three days, when I removed the bandage to clean the site, it was near impossible to keep the tubing from being pulled just a little farther from its original placement. Consequently, over time my vein started to show signs of damage. All these issues would have been minor if the PICC line was going to be very temporary, as PICC lines in the arm apparently are. There were no signs, however, that the Lyme disease was being eradicated, so this intravenous from of treatment would need to continue for many more months and possibly even years.

A few months later, while meeting with Rebecca, I shared my concerns and frustrations about the situation. As always, she listened and sympathized, and after looking at the line herself, she agreed the method was no longer appropriate. She suggested, however, that intravenous medication could still be administered, albeit in a different manner. She explained that the PICC line didn't have to be inserted in my arm; it could be inserted through my chest instead by having it inserted right into my heart through a device called a catheter.

When someone suggests your health can be improved by inserting a foreign object directly into your heart, it really makes you stop and think. *Is this worth it? What are the risks, really?* We trusted Rebecca completely, so neither Mary nor I had severe misgivings. Still, I would be dishonest if I said it didn't cause me to really stop and think. In the end, it was clear that if I wanted to move forward with antibiotic treatment, I really had no other choice.

Mary called the local hospital the next day and once again was happy to find someone there who could perform this procedure for me. The physician was even part of our healthcare network, so our insurance would cover it. Being able to schedule an appointment in only a few weeks' time was icing on the cake.

We were told that inserting a catheter into one's heart was a pretty routine operation and that it wouldn't even take very long to accomplish. I arrived at the hospital early in the morning, donned a gown, and was shown to a bed. About thirty minutes before it was my turn with the surgeon, I was anesthetized. Then, when I was fully under, the surgeon made a small incision in my chest wall, through which he threaded a line of tubing until it extended directly into a vein that led into my heart. He then placed a small catheter near the incision itself—a pincushion of sorts through which I would administer the liquid antibiotics—and finished by stitching the incision closed. When I woke from the anesthesia, I was told that I was wheeled back to the recovery room less than thirty minutes after having left.

The first thing I noticed, however—before I even opened my eyes—was searing pain; my neck and shoulder were on fire. When I told the nursing staff of my discomfort, I was repeatedly reassured that what I was feeling was normal and the pain I felt would slowly dissipate in the coming twelve to twenty-four hours. I suppose they work with people with various levels of tolerance for pain and were assuming that I was one of those who had very little. With all I'd been through on the farm as a kid, and as an adult with health problems for as long as I could remember, I was pretty sure my tolerance level was pretty high. Even so, I tried to bite my tongue and be patient, just as they'd asked, as I waited and waited for the pain to alleviate. If anything, though, it only seemed to intensify. I was relieved that a home health care nurse had been scheduled to come to our house within a few days to check the wound and show me how to insert the medicine.

Perhaps she'd be more responsive to my concerns and could give me some helpful insight into the situation.

When the nurse finally arrived, one of the first things out of my mouth was that the pain I was feeling was still pretty severe. Since by this time it had been a few days since the procedure, she told me that any continued discomfort at this point was not to be expected, yet cautioned that everyone reacts differently to medical procedures, so this could be completely normal as well. There wasn't much more to be said at that point, so she began to examine the wound and describe the process for administering the medication, which was the reason for her visit. She assured me it would be easy: I would simply poke the needle, which contained the antibiotic, through the skin into the pincushion-like device that had been inserted there.

After explaining the process, the nurse began to demonstrate it to us. She prepared the syringe, used her fingers to find the catheter, and inserted the needle into it. As she began to push the plunger, however, in an attempt to inject the medication, she began to look a little perplexed. After a moment or two of wiggling the syringe and feeling around with her fingers, and looking more closely at the insertion site, she was finally able to advance the plunger on the syringe so that the medication could be pushed into the line. The agony I felt as she did so was immediate. I clenched my jaw and stiffened my body in response to the pain, signs she definitely recognized but didn't seem to know how to address. She probably thought I simply had no pain tolerance whatsoever. Nonetheless, at the same time, she couldn't deny that it had not been easy to administer the medication, that something was at least a little off about the whole thing.

After seeing her struggle to perform the task, Mary and I couldn't help but wonder how either of us would be able to perform a task with which a trained and experienced nurse had such difficulty. It was difficult not to feel overwhelmed—not just by the responsibility but also (and perhaps even more so) by the pain.

When I woke up the next morning, my arm hurt more than ever. I went to work that day but could only use my right arm. Anything that required movement on the left side of my body where the catheter and line had been inserted was simply too painful. I was slightly encouraged that my arm seemed to feel a little better by the end of the day and considered that perhaps all of the nurses were right—that the discomfort really would decrease over time. So when it was time for me to give myself my first solo injection, I was starting to consider that this really could be done. I sat myself comfortably in a chair, wiped the area with antiseptic cleaner, and prepared the syringe. I used my fingers to locate the insertion area and tried to poke the needle through the skin. Mary and I found ourselves doing just as the nurse had done herself: we wiggled and readjusted and visually examined and then reexamined the location, then wiggled and felt some more. Eventually, I was able to force the needle into the catheter. Once there, I slowly wiggled and twisted and turned the syringe some more in an attempt to be able to push the plunger to dispense the medication.

After a considerable amount of time and effort, I was able to push some of the medication into my body, but as I struggled to do so, I noticed an unusual swelling under the skin around the insertion site. It appeared to me the medication was going beneath the skin and pooling there rather than flowing into the tube on its way to my heart. As I contemplated the situation, the pain slowly and steadily returned. Soon it was almost unbearable. I removed the needle and gingerly tried to move my arm and shoulder as if loosening up the area would relieve the pain. It didn't.

I would have liked to lay down and rest a bit, put some ice on the area to relieve some of the pain, and put something funny on TV to take my mind off the situation. It was Little League night, however, and as the head coach of my son's team, I needed to be with him on the field. The game would start within the hour, and we were already a little late to get going, so I'd just have to deal with this after the game. With little time to spare, I called my son, grabbed our gloves and bags, and headed to the diamond.

As soon as the last player left the dugout after the game, Mary and I jumped into the car and drove straight to the local hospital. We explained the situation to the nurse at the front desk, who listened politely, but clearly didn't believe what we were telling her. Eventually, we were shown to an examination room, where we were asked to wait for the nurse and doctor on call.

We told our story once again when the on-call nurse appeared. She, too, tried to hide a sigh as she filled a syringe with saline

Dangers of the Heart

and tried to inject it into the catheter to prove me wrong. Within seconds it was clear she was having the same difficulty the home health care nurse and I had experienced. I couldn't help feeling a little satisfaction when I noticed her forehead wrinkle into a frown while she tried to wiggle the needle and force the liquid into the line.

Eventually, she removed her gloves and left the room, returning a few minutes later with another nurse. The two of them took turns pushing and squeezing and repositioning the needle until, finally, they were able to insert some of the saline. Sure enough, the skin around the injection site began to swell as if the liquid was trapped beneath it. There were very few words between them and none toward us. We could see the confusion on their faces. They were still wearing the expression when the doctor arrived.

After a quick synopsis of their own experience, the doctor gave them his own *I don't really believe that* look and took a try himself. Once again, after considerable pushing and wiggling, he was able to insert some of the liquid, only to see it puddling beneath the surface of the skin. It took all the restraint I had to keep from smirking an *"I told you so"* to the experts.

The doctor turned to face us. "The medication," he said, "is not going into the line but is instead puddling beneath the surface of my skin." *Oh, really?* I thought. *Wow, imagine that!* "Don't attempt any more injections until you're able to see the surgeon who installed the catheter," he said. He then stated that there was really nothing more he could do and left the room.

When I called the surgeon the next morning, the receptionist was polite but seemingly unmoved by our plight. She told us the surgeon was at the clinic only once a week and had already been there that week, so I would have to wait until the following week to talk with him. This meant I would have to endure several more days of intense shoulder pain and use only one arm until he could see me. *Sure. No problem.*

After a difficult week, my appointment with the surgeon finally arrived. We were thrilled to be approaching what we hoped would be the end of this painful road and hopped enthusiastically out of our chairs when the nurse called our name. The doctor's first words were, "Why have you come to see me?" I told him what had occurred at home and again at the emergency room, but he seemed confused. It made sense when he interrupted me at one point to tell us he hadn't felt it necessary to read any of the notes in my file. So Mary and I began to retell the story, concluding with how it seemed like the liquid was gathering beneath the skin rather than passing through the tube. His only response was a firm, "This is impossible."

The surgeon filled a syringe with saline solution, and we watched him struggle to get to the point where the liquid pooled beneath the skin. Only then did he acknowledge there was something wrong. Boy, I had to hold my tongue. After a minute or so of closer investigation, the surgeon told us the catheter was malfunctioning and would need to be removed. *Oh great*, I thought. I was going to have to take another day off of work, undergo sedation again, and have to wait another week or so for it to take place. Just as this unpleasant scenario began to really sink in, though, the doctor pulled out a scalpel, some numbing solution, and some gauze and began making an incision in my skin. In only a few seconds, he pulled out the tube. Well, part of it, anyway. The whole thing didn't actually all come out—just the first seven inches or so. The rest, another two or three inches of tubing, was apparently still somewhere inside my chest.

Up to this point, the surgeon had maintained his cold, stone-faced demeanor, but his reaction to the less-than-whole piece of tubing pulling out brought about a bit of a change. He actually appeared a bit concerned. I'm sure he was trying not to show it, but it was impossible not to see he knew this could be a big problem. Even if we didn't know all the implications of the situation, we could tell by his loss of composure that it wasn't good.

The doctor quickly called the radiology department and made arrangements to have pictures taken of my chest. Someone was already waiting for me when I arrived. *Wow. This was, by far, the fastest I have ever been attended to at any hospital,* I thought, biting my nails. In only a few minutes, X-rays had been taken, and we were soon back downstairs in a waiting room across from the nurse's station. With the door slightly ajar, we heard the phone ring and saw the surgeon summoned to take the call. There was quite a bit of conversation, though it was difficult to follow what was being said. Eventually, the surgeon himself returned and brought us back into the original consultation room.

We were barely seated when the doctor showed us the images taken by the X-ray technician. He pointed out where my heart was and then highlighted the three-inch piece of tubing stuck inside it. Then, as if we hadn't already deduced it, the doctor explained the situation was not a good one. The piece of tubing had to be removed as soon as possible. If it moved—on its own or during the removal process—*it could be fatal.* He wasn't quite sure, though, how, when or where this would be done, so he sent us to wait in a nearby room once again as he went into his office to make some phone calls. I looked at Mary and could only shake my head. I tried to avoid pessimism, but once again, it dawned on me that this was just one more of the many events in my life that seemed to be part of a never-ending cruel series of jokes.

After a long thirty minutes of waiting, we heard the phone ring and noticed the surgeon was summoned once again. Moments later, he came into the waiting room and told us that a specialist was waiting for us at a larger clinic nearly an hour away and that upon my arrival, the emergency staff there would prepare me for immediate surgery to remove the piece of plastic tubing from my heart.

Mary drove and we talked about everything except what scared us most. We discussed the baseball game, what the kids were doing, and of course, the surgeon we'd met with that day. It was interesting to notice how his assured attitude had changed to how he acted when he sent us on our way; how the cocky man's smug expression had turned into actually showing a bit of compassion, concern, and outright fear. We might have felt just a bit sorry for him if we weren't so concerned about the outcome ourselves. As we neared the hospital, we mentally prepared ourselves for what was ahead, steeling ourselves for all that could possibly go wrong.

When we arrived at the hospital emergency room, we were asked to sit in the waiting room until the surgeon arrived. Within the hour, my name was called, and Mary and I were led into another series of rooms in preparation for the surgery. The doctor arrived shortly after we were settled, and he got right down to business. He explained the plan and didn't sugarcoat what could go wrong. They were going to cut a slit in my side and go up through a vein using a long line with a clamp at the end of it, and then the line would be inserted all the way into my heart. Once there, he would clamp onto the piece of tubing and carefully pull it out of the heart and back through the vein. The plan, of course, would change if he wasn't able to retrieve the piece of tubing using the method he had in mind.

It all sounded like a pretty incredible feat, yet, somehow, I wasn't worried at all—whether it could be removed or not. I had come to accept life or death for myself long ago. In some ways, I had also been looking for a way out of my miserable existence. *Maybe this is it,* I thought, dissociated from the situation. Still, I knew Mary was very worried, and it worried me—for her and our kids, and, of course, I thought of little Ferdie. I knew Mary would never be able to adopt him if I was gone. I wanted to be sure they would be okay, but it was a little late for that now.

Mary was shown to a small room where she would wait for a phone call from the nurse, who would call her right from the operating room when there was something significant to report. I was asked to put on a gown and lie in bed as the nurse began to talk with me about the procedure. She began by telling me that I would not be anesthetized for surgery but instead would be fully awake through it all. I wonder if she saw me shake my head in disbelief. Would this day—would my life—ever be short of shocking surprises?

Chapter 22

God's Love Provides

*But seek first His kingdom and His righteousness,
and all these things will be provided to you.*
Matthew 6:33

As I lay on the bed waiting for the offending piece of tubing to be removed, trying to put the worst-case scenario out of my mind, the nurse, perhaps making small talk because she could see I was nervous, asked if anything interesting had happened in my life recently. "As a matter of fact, something wonderful just happened the other day," I said with a smile. Two weeks earlier, our family had gone to a celebrity baseball game featuring players from our favorite football team, the Green Bay Packers. It was something my young son, Stephen, had wanted to experience for several years. After the game, we stuck around for a bit so he and his older brother, Joe, could try to get an autograph from the main celebrity, Donald Driver. Donald was the celebrity in charge of the event and the star receiver on our favorite NFL football team. As I stood along the first base line, I smiled as Stephen made his way back to me, carrying the football helmet he'd brought along. As if I couldn't tell from the smile on his face, I saw he'd achieved his goal: to have it signed by Mister Driver himself.

As Stephen and I stood admiring the autograph, we noticed a growing commotion just a few yards away. Fans had gathered, awaiting Donald Driver's exit from the stadium through the dugout. We quickly moved over to the group, where he was already waving to the onlookers, and we both waved back enthusiastically. Then, Donald took off a wristband and shot it into the crowd, followed by another wristband and then his hat. By this time, both of us were leaning against the back of the dugout near where he was standing in an attempt to be one of the lucky ones to snag one of his souvenirs. Surprisingly, he wasn't done yet. Donald bent over, untied a shoe, and threw it into the crowd opposite where we were standing. Then he threw his other shoe—in our direction—right to Stephen!

Stephen's eyes lit up with joy as the shoe fell into his hands. It was fully and clearly in his possession, and he could hardly believe it. As these things go, though, there were others nearby who were also hungry for such a treasure, including a lady (twice his size and at least three times his age). She was standing right beside him and was thrilled to be so close to such an opportunity and wasn't afraid to fight for what she wanted. Before Stephen fully realized what was happening, the woman snatched the shoe from his hands and ran away with it, waving it above her head in celebration of her good fortune. Stephen just stood there staring at her, shocked and disappointed. So close and yet so far!

Almost as quickly as it had begun, the hubbub died away after Donald Driver disappeared into the dugout. We'd probably have exited ourselves if we weren't still so shocked and disappointed by what had just occurred. Nevertheless, we took comfort in the fact that no matter how we felt that we'd lost out on an awesome opportunity, we'd actually already had one. It had been a wonderful day. The weather had been perfect, the game had been exciting, and we'd been able to see some of our favorite sports stars up close—or closer than ever before, anyway. It was such a fun experience.

So, after a few minutes of conversation about the situation, we began to gather our things. As we walked out of the stadium, we took one more look at the field and reminisced about "the one that got away." Only a few reporters and cameramen remained on the field. They noticed us, and one in particular called out to Stephen. "We saw what happened," the man said. "That just wasn't right." We spoke to them for a few minutes, during which one of them asked for our phone number in case they were able to find a way to resolve the situation. Mary jotted it on the back of an old program and tossed it down to them. Then we thanked them for their support, gave them a quick wave goodbye, and headed up the stairs to the nearest exit.

We hadn't even left the parking lot when Mary received a phone call from the reporter. He told us that he'd talked to a few people and was on the trail of setting things straight. He sure was. By the time we arrived home less than an hour later, news of "the shoe thief" was all over social media, and Mary had fielded phone calls from numerous local news reporters about the event. Amazingly, the story wasn't confined to just a few friends and reporters in the area: it was huge!

By the time Stephen's head hit the pillow the next night, he'd been contacted for interviews by newspapers, radio stations, and television channels all over the country—the story was in newspapers and on social media all over the world.

As if being interviewed by reporters all over the country wasn't overwhelming enough, imagine how Stephen felt when Donald Driver appeared out of the blue during one of them to gift him with a shoe personally—and another shoe, and a baseball bat, and books, all autographed by the one and only Donald Driver. Of course, even more exciting than the gifts, Stephen actually got to be the focus of Donald's attention, kind words, and smile, which was priceless.

The entire event had been such a blessing. It had brought such joy and pleasure to Stephen's life and, at the same time, had given Stephen the opportunity to model forgiveness and compassion. When others goaded him to be critical and angry at the woman who had taken the shoe, Stephen responded time after time with kindness and understanding. We couldn't have been more proud and humbled by his godliness. What an amazing, amazing gift.

I finished recounting the story to the medical staff just as I heard the surgeon announce, "Here it is!" It was incredible to think that the chunk of plastic he held in his forceps had so recently been lodged deep in my heart, and I was greatly relieved to still be alive. I was thankful that my family would now be able to feel some peace and definitely happiness, too, that I'd be able to see them all again.

As I was wheeled to the recovery room, I couldn't help but wonder if it had truly been just a coincidence that the nurse had asked me if anything exciting had happened recently in my life and if perhaps our recent bit of excitement with Donald Driver might have been one of God's blessings sent to help us through this difficult time. It certainly would be easy to overlook the situation, as I'd likely done so many other times when He had brought good things to me. Our family had been buoyed by an unexpected series of joys that had sustained us during an unexpected series of trials, and I suddenly felt overwhelmed by God's immeasurable mercy and love.

Although the immediate danger had passed, I now faced a tough question: Should I get a new catheter inserted and begin this process all over again, or had this experience been a sign that it wasn't a good idea? I certainly hadn't yet been healed from the chronic Lyme disease, so I needed to do something. For lack of another option, I decided to give the intravenous antibiotic another try. I called the original surgeon to set up an appointment to have the catheter reinserted. The receptionist took my name and told me she'd call me back after talking with the doctor. Within a few hours, she called me back. To my utter amazement, she told me that neither the original surgeon nor his partner were willing to reinsert the tube. The receptionist relayed that neither of them, in fact, even believed that chronic Lyme disease actually existed, which ultimately made the procedure a pointless endeavor.

I shouldn't have been surprised to hear that the surgeons didn't believe I had chronic Lyme disease, and I should have been so accustomed to reaching dead ends that this shouldn't have been a big deal. Nonetheless, it was. Again and again, I faced roadblocks to overcome. Rather than feel protected and supported by medical professionals who were supposed to care about sick people, I felt manipulated and trapped by them time and time again. It was illogical and almost unbearable because each time, I felt adrift in a sea of unknowns that could so easily have been navigated if someone in the field would simply have given me a few thoughtful minutes of their time to help steer me in the right direction.

At this point in time, I couldn't see that the surgeons' refusals could be one more of God's blessings in disguise, but it very likely was because I soon located a surgeon at another nearby hospital who was willing to do the surgery. It was a routine procedure for him, actually, and he would not only be glad to do the procedure but would also be able to provide me with a more effective type of device than the one that had been installed in me previously. The Groshong Catheter, as it is called, is easier for the patient to manage, more durable, and costs about the same as the previous catheter. We were convinced and impressed. This guy clearly knew what he was doing.

The procedure was quick and painless, and injecting my medicine worked the first time without a hitch. As you can imagine, however, this latest turn of health events had taken another large bite out of our already-tight budget. Moreover, the timing was particularly precarious because, in addition to the expenses of my many past medical issues, we had a big expense on the horizon in the form of travel to Africa, where we'd finally meet and bring home our new son.

Travel plans for our trip to Africa were complicated. We didn't have much padding in our savings account, so it would be fiscally conservative for just one of us to make the journey. A trip to Africa, however, was a once–in–a–lifetime experience. Furthermore, since it was the homeland of our newest family member, it seemed important for all of us to experience what Ferdie's life had been like there, as well as for Ferdie to know we could relate to his life at least a little because we'd seen even a small part of it.

After considerable discussion and prayer, we decided to shoot for the moon. We'd all go to Africa—even if we had to borrow the money to do so. Some things are just more important than money.

As the months passed, I learned how to adapt my life to accommodate my new catheter. Praise God that it worked so well from the start! The antibiotics, however, seemed to make little difference to my health since I felt neither better nor worse. The catheter was a constant commitment and reminder of my health challenges. Still, thoughts about my health took a back seat to my preoccupation about what lay ahead in our lives with our new son.

The timing of our trip to Africa initially appeared to be perfectly timed with the kids' summer vacation, which would have been very convenient. As we'd discovered so many times before, however, the African adoption timeline is full of unforeseen starts and stops that can and often do change plans by days or even months at a time. It seemed that every time we heard from Ruth, our liaison at the orphanage, there was one crazy delay or another. First, our documents were returned because of missing signatures and errors in translation. Then, the country's legal workforce began a several-week hiatus due to a national holiday. Eventually, just when it seemed like everything was finally in place, Ruth contacted us to say there was yet another issue—one with the potential to derail the adoption altogether.

Ferdie's biological father, who had passed away several years before, had signed the required documents allowing Ferdie's adoption. His biological mother, however, who was still living, hadn't done so. The judge was obviously not comfortable with this situation and ruled that the mother must first be found, questioned, and asked to either sign paperwork to release him to the custody of the court or to assume responsibility for Ferdie herself. The usually rock-steady Ruth seemed unnerved about this, which made us anxious. It was hard to comprehend that we were now faced with the possibility of not being able to adopt Ferdie after all. We had truly grown to love this fresh-faced, smiling boy and, at this point, could not imagine life without him.

Then something inside me shifted as I remembered how clearly God moved upon me when I saw Ferdie's face on Mary's computer screen. I remembered the love I felt and knew in my heart that God is love (1 John 4:8) and love never fails (1 Corinthians 13:8). I suddenly realized with certainty that God was in control and that things would happen in His timing, according to His will. We realized God would do what He said He would do, so we prayed, waited, and tried to be okay with whatever God had planned.

Several weeks passed as we waited to hear news from Africa. Would Ferdie's biological mother be found? If she was, would she sign the papers, or would she want to care for Ferdie herself? If she wasn't found, would the judge be willing to allow Ferdie to be adopted without her signature? Ruth told us Ferdie's lawyer was of the opinion everything would be okay, but she didn't seem so sure of this herself.

God's Love Provides

As we waited, I began to ponder God's love. For years, I've meditated on the well-known Bible verse that tells me to love God with all my heart, soul, mind, and might (Luke 10:27). I never had a hard time understanding the fact that I was to use all of my heart, soul or mind to love God, but how in the world was I to love Him with all of my might? The task seemed impossible—or at least way beyond my capabilities. I wasn't even sure what it meant. Was I supposed to sit at a table and focus on Him with extreme intensity until I passed out? Maybe I should gnash my teeth and squint my eyes while envisioning Him, trying to squeeze love for Him almost physically out of my heart. Or perhaps I was to put my physical capabilities to the test through strict fasting or by carrying a replica of Jesus' cross while on my own trek through the city.

As hard as I tried, I just couldn't comprehend how to love God with all of my might. Then one day, I saw a news program featuring amazing achievements by ordinary people around the world. As I watched, my eyes began to tear up. These were not tears of sadness but of amazement at the love and power of God, who had caused all of these incredible things to occur. It made my heart swell for Him. I pondered these things for several days after, and I slowly began to recognize that in those moments, as in so many others throughout my life, the feeling in my heart was one of deep love for my God. My tears had been a sign of the awe I felt for His love, power, and greatness. At that moment, I recognized that I did know what it felt like to love God with all of my might because I was doing just that—and in fact, I had been doing so for a very long time.

On November 20, 2011, early in the morning, Mary opened an email from Ruth. In it, she explained the weeks of searching had proven fruitless—the authorities were never able to find Ferdie's mother. Subsequently, the judge approved Ferdie's release to be adopted, and the adoption was moving forward again. It was done! Ferdie was officially our son!

Of course, once we received that news, we wanted to leave as soon as possible to meet Ferdie and bring him home with us. Ruth, however, quickly told us we would have to wait until *early January* to fetch him. *Are you kidding?* I thought as my heart dropped. January was an eternity away, and our daughter

Julia had been cast in the high school musical to be performed in early February. If we left in January, she would have to give up her role in the musical. Her role hadn't been selected yet, so we didn't know if it was to be a starring feature or something inconsequential. She had always dreamed of having the starring part in the play, and now, being a high school senior, if ever there was a chance for this to occur, it would be that year. We couldn't take it away from her, but we also didn't want to have to wait a month longer than the eternity it seemed we already had to wait. It was an extremely difficult decision.

After a lot of prayer and consideration, we decided to wait until after Julia's performance. This, in fact, turned out to be a blessing in disguise as we didn't realize we'd need the extra time to prepare for our trip and the coming change in our family. We were excited but also uncertain, and before we knew it, it was February 12, 2012: time for us to board the plane for Africa!

In addition to our own belongings, we'd been asked to take about eighty pounds of dry baby formula that had been donated to the orphanage by a small group somewhere in the United States. The group had contacted Mary asking if we would take the baby formula with us to save the cost of shipping. Mary agreed without hesitation; it was a small way we could say thanks to the Lord for what He was giving us. The formula was delivered to us packed in plastic Ziploc bags, maybe three pounds apiece, with a piece of red tape over the seal to prevent any spills. The airline allotted two pieces of luggage each, but since we didn't need that much, we split the baby formula among four different duffel bags and added them to our luggage.

It felt so good to be able to help, and it really didn't inconvenience us. It wasn't until I was loading our luggage into the car, however, that I realized the duffel bags and their contents had a remarkable resemblance to contraband and wondered if this could cause us some serious trouble. I hadn't felt the need to test it, but surely it really *was* baby formula. I had been so distracted by everything else I just hadn't thought of it until it was too late to do anything about it.

It was an interesting feeling leaving the house, knowing upon our return that our lives would be changed forever. Thankfully, our trip to Chicago was much less eventful than our last drive to an airport had been all those years ago. No one threw up, and we were extra careful to turn all the lights out when we parked the car at the airport.

Finally, it was time. We were going to Africa! Awaiting us was the continent of sun and sand and all kinds of animals we had only seen in zoos and books. It was so much bigger than that, though, because we were going to meet a boy who had known only that land and its people for all of his thirteen years. He would call us "Dad" and "Mom," and we would call him our son.

After an eight-hour flight, we landed in Brussels, Belgium, where we had a three-hour layover. We then boarded again for a six-hour flight to Ouagadougou, Burkina Faso. It had been a very long day, and while everyone was in good spirits, we were all eager to arrive and disembark. Finally, we felt the landing gear meet the runway. Touchdown, Africa!

It was about 4:00 p.m. local time when we arrived in Ouagadougou. The first thing I noticed stepping out of the plane was the glorious, wonderful warmth of the African sun, *which was so much better than the one-degree Fahrenheit weather we had left less than twenty-four hours earlier.* I looked around curiously and noticed this airport was far from the busy commercial zone we had experienced in Chicago or Brussels. Instead of the carpeted inner concourse leading from the plane to the building, I saw a tall set of metal stairs leading to the blacktop of the runway. Where in Chicago and Brussels there had been hundreds of busy travelers moving briskly to their destination, there now were a few dozen of us slowly meandering our way to the checkpoint.

The security personnel at the airport were obviously less excited to see us than we were to see them. Their ordinary afternoon at work was a once-in-a-lifetime opportunity for us. We couldn't understand the French signs and instructions, so we just followed the other passengers. Soon we were standing in front of an austere security guard seated in a small booth. He gestured at us impatiently, then stamped our passports and shooed us away.

As we approached the baggage claim area, a man in military garb, carrying a huge rifle and a long knife on his belt, seemed to be the official baggage checker. Suddenly my stomach lurched. I hadn't given much thought to the duffel bags since we left, but *what* if it *wasn't baby* formula in those packages, after all? I tried to remain calm and smiling, handing him our luggage. After a cursory examination of the contents of the suitcases, he pushed them back at us without concern, but then he turned toward the duffel bags. *Oh boy.* I thought. *Here we go.* When he unzipped the first duffel bag and looked inside, I thought his eyes were going to jump out of his head. He quickly snatched up one of the baggies and barked some orders to four other soldiers standing nearby. They instantly marched over to us, clutching their rifles menacingly.

Chapter 23

Strangers in a Strange Land

For the whole Law is fulfilled in one word, in the statement, "You shall love your neighbor as yourself."
Galatians 5:14

We were soon surrounded by the soldiers. The leader reached for the long knife that was holstered to his belt and made some sharp pronouncements to his colleagues in a language we couldn't understand. He then slit one of the plastic baggies open and pushed his knife into the powder to extract a bit. I wanted to shout an explanation of the situation, to tell the men I was just doing someone a favor and was just carrying a load of baby formula. I felt compelled to protest that I was completely innocent of anything bad—if there was anything bad involved. I knew the soldiers couldn't understand me, however, and even if they could, they probably wouldn't believe me. So I just stood and watched, knowing that if those baggies were filled with something nefarious, we were all in serious trouble.

The soldier raised his knife to his tongue and looked up and away, carefully considering the message from his taste buds. His face puckered briefly as if the taste wasn't what he'd been expecting. Then, without much ado, he grunted a few words to his companions and waved us through to the exit. Just like that, my visions of twenty years to life in a dank foreign prison evaporated.

We all sighed a deep breath of relief, gave the soldiers a weak smile, gathered the rest of our belongings, and headed brusquely toward the exit.

Crisis averted, we focused our attention on the next challenge at hand: finding Ruth, a woman we'd never met in a country far, far from home. For some reason, neither party had specified exactly where to meet, so we decided to just take a seat on a long wooden bench near what we surmised was the main doorway. It was a pleasant break from the hustle and bustle we'd experienced in the past hour or so and gave us a great opportunity to take in the sights and sounds of this new land.

It was impossible not to be inspired by the energy around us. Just outside the building where we'd sat, a group of African men were singing, dancing, and playing their drums. We later learned that the commotion was a celebration of Burkina Faso's second-place finish in the African Nations Cup soccer tournament. The entire country had been celebrating this achievement. Schools and businesses had been closed for days to enable workers, students, teachers, and shoppers an opportunity to fully appreciate the event. Although the tournament had ended the day before, there was still excitement in the air.

The joy on the faces around us was contagious, and we soon found ourselves deep in appreciation of our surroundings, so it was almost a surprise when we eventually saw Ruth and her ever-present smile heading our way. It's an odd feeling to meet someone in person that you've communicated with so extensively yet had never met. One doesn't know whether to act as old friends or new acquaintances. After a somewhat awkward greeting and a bit of small talk, she suggested that we head out on our way.

Not knowing where we were headed, we simply followed Ruth across the dusty gravel parking lot, apparently toward her vehicle. It was curious that with each step, we gained additional individuals to our party, which Ruth didn't even seem to notice. By the time we arrived at her SUV, a small group of smiling, enthusiastic young men had gathered around us. As if it had been previously planned, a few of them began to toss a rope to the top of the car while others began to shimmy up to the roof, then reach down for our bags. Ahhh. Now I saw. The men had come with us to help us load our baggage and, upon doing so, would be financially reimbursed for their efforts. It was easy to see how much Ruth appreciated the young mens' industriousness, and it caused me to reflect upon how different this was from what I'd been accustomed to in America. It was the first of many such realizations.

Once our baggage was firmly fastened to the roof of our vehicle, Ruth got behind the steering wheel, started the engine, and headed out of the parking lot onto the road, where we immediately became ensnared in the chaos of traffic of Ouagadougou. Bicycles, mopeds, and cars swarmed around us like bees en route to the juiciest flowers. There didn't seem to be any rhyme or reason to their movement; everyone moved as he or she individually desired without regard to a particular lane or speed. I was amazed that Ruth didn't seem fazed by the commotion. She confidently maneuvered through the crowded streets without running anyone over—or allowing them to run us over. I was especially intrigued by the many people who were zipping around on their mopeds. They seemed able to weave in and out without much hindrance from the million and a half others who called this city their home. It looked very freeing, despite the fact that the potential for imminent danger seemed extremely high.

In addition to the fact that it's generally not safe to travel through the countryside after dark in Burkina Faso, because Ruth did so much adoption-related business in the capital city, it made sense for her to have a place to stay while there. She actually shared it with a foreign couple who spent considerable time there as volunteers who maintained wells all over the country. It was to this house that we were currently headed, and Ruth, despite the chaos around us, was fully in charge behind the wheel. The trip was fascinating in every way: unique sights, sounds, and smells were everywhere. Eventually, Ruth turned off the busy road to one that was slightly quieter and then another that was even quieter still. She soon paused in front of a tall, closed gate, honked her horn, and waited a few minutes until the gate was opened from the inside by someone she'd obviously expected to be there. She then pulled into the short driveway and stopped beside a small, quaint residence.

Once we'd untethered our luggage from the vehicle, Ruth showed us to our rooms and invited us to make ourselves at home while she took care of some business on her laptop. It was definitely refreshing to sit for a few minutes and catch our bearings. Still, at the same time, it was hard to sit inside knowing that there was a world just outside the gate that was full of life—a life full of curiosities and wonders I'd not yet had an opportunity to experience. I just had to check it out.

I spent most of our first evening sitting beside the street in front of the home where we were staying, just watching the mopeds buzzing around in the warm evening. Of course, there were plenty of other things to see, too. People who weren't on mopeds were conversing as they walked in pairs or small groups down the road, and a small group of children were playing soccer on the field across the street. It didn't take long for my heart to warm to everything around me. In Ouaga, I saw what life without easy access to TV and other electronic devices would be like: more time to talk, play, or even just take a walk. It was very refreshing.

It probably sounds strange, but I felt at home in Ouagadougou almost right away. Ruth's hospitality was likely responsible for a great deal of my satisfaction, but there was more to it than that. It was so wonderful to be in a slower-paced environment without the constant distraction of technology. It was so much more calm here in Ouaga. The crazy buzz that typically would fill the air around me was gone. As a result, it was easier for me to focus on the people, the scenery, and my own thoughts. There was also the weather! We'd left wintry Wisconsin, full of cloudy skies, snow, and cold winds, but here all I felt was the continual hug of the warm sunshine, which felt absolutely heavenly.

Despite how great it felt in Africa, there was one big problem: we couldn't speak the language. Consequently, it was extremely difficult to communicate with the lovely people around us. Sure, I could smile and throw a "Bonjour!" at the people around me, but I wanted to do more than that. Everyone was so friendly and seemed to jump at the chance to help us whenever they could. I wanted each of them to know how much I appreciated that and how much I'd loved to have had the chance to really get to know them.

At nightfall, I returned to the house and conversed with Ruth. I had so many questions. We talked about the people of Burkina Faso and their customs, about the children and the orphanage, and of course, about Ferdie. We were finally so close to meeting our son. Every so often, I felt like I might have to pinch myself—I could hardly believe I was sitting in a home in Africa with my family, talking with a wonderful woman about a child she'd helped raise who was now our own.

After a very cozy night at Ruth's house, we awoke to the chatter of children playing football in the field across the street. Ruth had left to get breakfast and run a few errands, so it was just our family in the residence. We weren't sure what time she would be back, so Mary, the kids, and I took a walk down the street while we waited. It was obviously just another day for the many men, women, and children we passed, some on their mopeds, some sitting or standing by their wares along the street, and others doing business in their small shops. They all smiled at us and tried to converse, but all we could do was wave and smile back.

After our excursion, we headed back to the house for breakfast. I'd brought a few bags of quinoa, which was one of the only things I'd been able to eat at home with minimal reaction, so I boiled some water and cooked it on the stove in the tiny kitchen. Mary and the kids sat at the table and talked, played cards, or did some of the homework they'd brought along while they awaited Ruth's return. We were blessed enough to have internet access at Ruth's house, so the kids also checked in on things at home—despite the fact that today was still yesterday for those we knew there, and all their friends and family in the U.S. were fast asleep.

Before long, Ruth arrived with loaves of freshly baked French bread that smelled divine. Our breakfast time was marred, however, by Ruth's concern over trouble she'd had with her vehicle while on her errands. In the end, it was decided that if she could just get the engine to start, it would likely be good to go and could be fixed upon our return to the orphanage. So after eating and tidying up, we took our bags to the truck. Unfortunately, the engine wouldn't start with a simple turn of the key, so Ruth put it into neutral, guided it down the driveway, and enlisted some passersby to give it a push-start. It was definitely an unconventional way to start the final leg of our journey, but this was an unconventional journey—so why not?

As she'd done so well the day before, Ruth plowed the vehicle through the swarm of mopeds and maze of roads in the city until we arrived at what appeared to be a security checkpoint of some kind on the outskirts of town. Ruth slowed the vehicle and eventually came to a stop—without cutting the engine, of course, which would have made starting it once again a bit of an issue. Aside from the soldiers milling around, several women were sitting beside blankets upon which a variety of fresh fruit and vegetables had been placed. Some women wore a young child in a wrap upon their back while their older children called out to passersby to further encourage a sale. When two soldiers appeared beside the vehicle, Ruth rolled down her window to speak with them. We couldn't understand their exchange, but Ruth appeared unflustered, so it was apparent that this, too, was just another routine part of the travel process in Burkina Faso.

Ruth slowly accelerated away from the checkpoint, apparently unbothered by the numerous goats, chickens, and oxen walking beside (and occasionally across) the road. I'd grown up in Wisconsin, so I'd learned to keep an eye out for deer that might suddenly wander onto the pavement. Nevertheless, I'd never had to deal with such an assortment of wildlife in and near the thoroughfare in such numbers, so I was definitely impressed by Ruth's composure. Knowing how much damage a single deer could inflict on a vehicle, I was definitely hoping we'd not experience such a fate with something as sturdy as an ox.

After we'd traveled for several miles, Ruth asked if I'd like to drive for a while. I'd had a chance to get a feel for the road and any possible obstructions by then and felt I could handle it, so I eagerly agreed. Ruth pulled over to the side of the road, and we got out to exchange seats. Once seated behind the wheel, I adjusted the seat and briefly inspected the dials on the dashboard, then edged back onto the road. Ruth gave me a few tips about the driving protocol as I somewhat tentatively increased my speed. Apparently, there was no speed limit, but Ruth indicated that it was best to keep speeds much like we were familiar with at home—about 88-96 kilometers per hour (55-60 miles per hour). Any faster than that, and it would be nearly impossible to have enough time to react to other vehicles safely—and the occasional animal—on the narrow road.

In an hour or so, we were already nearing our destination of Yako. I pulled over to switch places once again with Ruth in preparation for the nearing checkpoint on the outskirts of the village, where we once again passed a small group of soldiers and women sitting along the road beside a spread of produce they wished to sell.

Although it was much smaller, the citizens of Yako resembled those we'd seen in Ouagadougou—at least to us. Perhaps it would be more accurate to say that they had more in common with the people of Ouaga than with their counterparts in America because, unlike what occurs in most American communities, the people in Burkina Faso spend most of their waking hours outside interacting with their friends and neighbors rather than hanging out by themselves in their homes or places of business for most of the day. Along the road, men gathered in groups in front of small shops. Some were conversing as they sipped their tea, while others stood beside an open grill, upon which chicken was being cooked for hungry passersby. A few shops featured men fixing bicycles or repairing mopeds. There were occasional larger structures inside which large bags of rice, beans, and other foodstuffs were sold, shops that advertised the sale of wigs, and buildings upon which beauticians invited customers to stop in to have their hair braided.

While the street itself was less chaotic than it had been in Ouagadougou, it was still a busy place full of bicyclists, mopeds, and people traveling by foot. Animals meandered, children ran, and women walked with babies wrapped in slings on their backs while carrying bowls or baskets of fruit on their heads. Donkeys pulled carts loaded with wares, and an occasional truck or small car dodged in and out of everything else that filled the streets. There was so much to see in every direction it was hard to decide where to look.

Knowing the orphanage was now only minutes away, our hearts beat faster in anticipation of the opportunity to finally meet our new son and brother. When we turned the last corner before the gates to the orphanage, we saw the brick wall that surrounded his home, and I tried to view it and the other surroundings the way Ferdie must have for most of his life. This was the neighborhood and the life he'd always known. It was his home, his place of safety and love. It was where he played with friends and learned the ways of the world. These were the walls that surrounded his bedroom, his school, and his soccer field. It was a little unnerving, yet extremely exciting.

When Ruth honked the horn at the gate, it was quickly opened by a young man from the inside. I'm not sure if he was there to protect the place or was just in charge of opening and closing the gate, but we would come to learn he, or someone else, was always there, waiting to do so. He waved as we drove in, and we eagerly waved back while Ruth drove across the full length of the courtyard. Our eyes curiously searched all corners of the area for the boy we had seen in the photos. Did Ferdie know we were coming? Was he waiting for us? Was he watching us from somewhere we couldn't see? Was he scared? Excited? Sad? Confused? Worried? Should we run up and hug him or stand back and give him some space? Would we be able to communicate with him, or would it just be a lot of pointing and smiling? Why hadn't we thought to ask Ruth about this earlier? What, exactly, was the plan for this momentous and yet completely unscripted occasion?

Once Ruth had driven across the length of the courtyard, she stopped the vehicle beneath an awning next to what appeared to be the building where we'd be staying. We tentatively opened the doors and exited, still scanning the surroundings for a boy who resembled the image in the pictures. It was a bit of a letdown to see no sign of anyone enthusiastically running toward us, but since we'd not discussed how our first meeting would take place, it wasn't too concerning. We knew Ruth had a plan and that no matter what, it wouldn't be long before we'd be face-to-face with our son.

The screen door closed behind us as we entered the small home only a few feet from the vehicle. There was a couch and several chairs around a TV to our right and a large dinner table surrounded by eight chairs straight ahead. Entries to three bedrooms on the left were mirrored on the right side of the building. Ruth told us this was where most of the missionaries stayed when they came to help for a while. To make room for our family, though, most of them had moved out and found alternative places to stay so our family could all be together. What kindness!

Ruth pointed Joe and Stephen to the room on the right, just past the TVs, suggested that Julia take the room in the far left corner, and guided Mary and me to the room in the nearest left corner of the building. We dispersed to our own areas with our luggage and returned quickly to the main room, where we took seats on the couch and chairs by the TV beside Ruth. Everything seemed to be in place. Almost everything, anyway: there was still no Ferdie. Ruth looked at us with a smile, which we nervously returned, and then asked us if we were ready to meet our son. We sure were!

Chapter 24

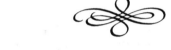

A Change of Season

*He predestined us to adoption as sons and
daughters through Jesus Christ to Himself,
according to the good pleasure of His will,
to the praise of the glory of His grace, with
which He favored us in the Beloved.*
Ephesians 1:5-6

Ruth sent someone to fetch Ferdie. I looked around the room as we waited. It felt surreal to be sitting in the room we'd longingly studied as we waited for the adoption to be finalized.

It wasn't long before the door opened and an adorable boy appeared. He stood for a moment, then tentatively entered the room. I'm sure it was more than a little intimidating for him, considering that the room was full of unknown faces, all staring directly at him. He walked slowly to Ruth and sat on her lap. Mary and I resisted our urge to run directly to him and wrap him in our arms, choosing instead to smile and utter a few words as a greeting. It dawned on both of us that we should have thought more about what would be appropriate in this situation—as if it were possible for such a thing to have been established. Since we hadn't, however, we simply deferred to our hostess, who definitely played her role as "Mama Ruth" in outstanding fashion.

Ruth started by speaking to Ferdie in French, then restating her words in English for the rest of us. She spoke briefly about who we were and what she had in mind for this first time together. She then turned to me and invited me to introduce myself to Ferdie, followed by the same from Mary and the kids. It was suddenly very obvious that while we had so much we wanted to say to him, this might be a time when fewer words would be best—as if he could understand any of them, anyway. So, in the end, we ended up just using big smiles and lots of hand gestures to try to communicate our excitement and the deep love we already felt for him. After even a short period of time, it was evident that this method of communication wasn't very satisfying nor sustainable, so it was a welcome relief when someone handed Ferdie a soccer ball, and he invited Joe and Stephen to go outside with him to play. They followed Ferdie eagerly, and the rest of us tumbled out of the house after them.

The orphanage was mostly surrounded by a tall stone wall, creating a large rectangular area. Several buildings took over as a border in places where the wall ended, such as rooms where the children slept and a few brick structures where the children attended class. The courtyard itself contained numerous elements: a sandy, well-used, and very small soccer field; a small health clinic; a women's weaving area; a baby enclosure and infant sleeping room; a water tower and playground equipment; an outhouse and shower area; several tables (many shaded by a thatched roof of sorts); a few water pumps; and two main cooking areas consisting of fire pits over which meals were served three times a day.

Thankfully, the courtyard also had a few trees in it, so we headed toward one that was beside the soccer field in hopes that it would keep the hot sun from our faces while we watched the boys play. We were almost immediately joined by a swarm of smiling young children, who eagerly shouted greetings and reached out to shake our hands. Meanwhile, on the soccer field, a crowd of older boys had already assembled themselves into two teams and were kicking the ball around amidst competitive cheers and jeers. I chuckled when I saw that Joe and Stephen had removed their shoes in an attempt to fit in with the rest of the bunch, for whom barefoot play was routine. While the others raced up and down and zig-zagged in and out after the ball and each other, Joe and

Stephen could only gingerly tiptoe across the hard ground. This was a cause for laughter from the boys on the field as well as those of us who watched. Their feet were clearly not as tough as the others, which made for quite a comical situation, even for the two of them.

Although it might initially appear that the soccer game was the main focus of everyone's attention, it was soon apparent that the gathering of children around Julia was equal in significance and size. Someone had brought some paper with them, and most of the kids used it to draw, write, or color while pleasantly chattering away as they did so. One girl, in particular, had found a position right next to Julia and was soon exchanging words and phrases with her, teaching Julia French words in exchange for their English counterparts. Her name, she said, was Fani. She was a few years younger than Julia and was obviously inquisitive, smart, and outgoing. She impressed us with her enthusiasm and her ready smile.

Occasionally, a child or two would approach Mary and me and tell us something in French. All we could do in return, though, was shrug our shoulders and display a look of confusion to indicate our disappointment that we didn't know what they were saying. They didn't seem to mind. Neither did we.

As I sat on the bench listening to the laughter of the boys on the field and the children beside us, I was suddenly overwhelmed by the relative strangeness of what was happening around me. I was on the same planet but in another world, and it was completely mind-boggling. Then I thought about Ferdie and how he might be feeling right now. I was immediately aghast that I'd never previously considered the situation from Ferdie's point of view. How selfish and inconsiderate I felt!

Did Ferdie really want to be adopted? Ruth had indicated he'd said he wanted a family on several occasions before, but now that it was happening, did he still feel that way? When he found out that we were the family that was interested in adopting him, was he still interested? Was he worried? Was he scared?

I also began to question the practicalities of our situation that I hadn't considered earlier. Were we going to be able to communicate with each other well enough to manage the essentials once back home, far away from anyone that could translate if needed? Would time away from his homeland cause Ferdie to lose comprehension of his own native language—and was that fair? Was there anything we could do to help him hang on to his language and culture when he was in a new land so far removed from it? These were some seriously big issues—too big to really understand myself and definitely too big for a twelve-year-old boy to have to face. What was the alternative, though? Was staying in the orphanage just so he could remain within the culture he grew up in a worthy trade-off?

While I sat pondering these complex issues, a noisy crescendo from the soccer field suddenly returned me to the present moment, where the voices of the victors from the morning's soccer match were mixed in with their opponents, who were just as excitedly protesting that the results weren't actually as they appeared. Despite the commotion, though, there wasn't a sad or angry face anywhere in the crowd. Rather, there were smiles all around, and even an occasional arm slung over the shoulder of another. My heart swelled with admiration for these boys as I imagined how differently I'd seen groups of American children responding at the end of a hard-played match, especially one that was unmonitored by adults or referees or any kind. It dawned on me that humanity really was capable of so much better than we often saw in our own land of abundance. It wouldn't be the last time during our stay in Africa that I'd recognize that true poverty is not about money. Rather, it is a condition in which the depletion of community and faith results in an existence that is neither truly joyful nor fulfilling, as is so often the case in countries like America, where the value of money has often been elevated beyond its true worth.

Eventually, the commotion died down and most dispersed to other areas of the orphanage. Ferdie and Ruth talked a bit, then he, too, headed back to his room to clean up for supper. Unbeknownst to us, some women had been preparing the evening's meal while we sat enjoying the sights and sounds outside, and all we needed to do was show up. Joe and Stephen had a bit of cleaning up to do before they were ready to enter the building, so they each took a quick rinse from the pump to take off the first layer of grime so they'd not make too much of a mess on their way to the shower inside. Mary, Julia, and I tried to make ourselves helpful by setting the table and assisting with any other small tasks. We soon realized, however, that the most helpful thing we could do was stay out of the way.

Before long, the food was on the table and everything appeared to be ready, so we each took a seat and looked expectantly at each other. We were all there—except for Ferdie. Come to think of it, Ferdie had been gone a surprisingly long time, and even Ruth commented that, given what she'd spoken with him about outside, he should have returned by now. Not wanting to begin without him, we all simply sat, smiling at each other, making rather awkward small talk. Eventually, we heard a knock on the door and were glad to see that Ferdie had returned. He'd been sent to simply wash off his feet but had instead taken a full shower so as to be completely refreshed and clean for dinner.

Our first meal together, while delicious, was rather uncomfortable because it was very confusing. Ferdie was now our son, so it seemed logical that it was now our responsibility to monitor his behaviors. Whoa, not so fast. The woman who'd assumed those responsibilities for the last seven years—the woman he'd come to love and trust and defer to as his parent of sorts—was still very much present in his life in general and in the very room, to be specific. To whom, then, should the authority belong? Further complicating this situation was the fact that we, as Americans, hadn't even a small awareness of behaviors that were and were not culturally appropriate at the dinner table in Burkina Faso. Therefore, our qualifications for this position were already severely limited. How, then, were we to proceed? Should we sit back and allow Ruth to take the lead, or should we jump right in with both feet and make comments and corrections as we saw fit along the way? It was definitely something that should have been considered before we'd found ourselves in this position, but as in so many other instances to come, we hadn't expected this unexpected, so all we could do was our very imperfect best.

Through gritted teeth and nervous banter, we clunked our way through the meal until it was finally over. As we finished helping clear the table, we both exhaled a sigh of relief—if only so we could stop the charade and take a break from each other and the serious tone we had added to dinner. Mary retreated to the bedroom and closed the door behind her. I collapsed into the easy chair by the window, recalling, for the first time in months, the words of our adoption consultant: "Older child adoption is not for the faint of heart." I was beginning to understand what she had meant, and we were only getting started.

After supper, we sat down together to watch a video on the TV in the main room. When it was bedtime, Joe, Stephen, and Ferdie headed into their rooms, Julia to hers, and Mary and I to ours. Mary and I finally had a few minutes alone to talk about the events of this momentous day. Mary began by sharing her discomfort around superseding Ruth's role as housemother. This led to her expressing concern about Ruth's impression of our parenting, which soon led to her sharing worries that Ferdie might be disappointed in us and, after getting to know us a bit, may not still wish to be part of our family. Like a speeding locomotive, she went on to talk about the stress she was feeling as a result of living in another's home, worrying about how the kids would get along now that Ferdie was in the mix, and fretting about how to help Ferdie see and understand our expectations without being offended by them. In the end, Mary confessed she just wanted to be home to deal with all that was happening, where she'd be free from some of the extraneous complications. There wasn't much I could do other than reassure her that she was doing great and remind her that God would take care of everything. Mary eventually stopped talking and simply turned away from me with tears running down her face. I held her tightly but knew my arms were of little consolation. The future was suddenly overwhelming, and there was absolutely nothing anyone could do to make it less so—except to trust in God. It was easy to say but so hard to do.

The next day, our family—Ferdie included—left the orphanage to drive back to Ouagadougou to take care of some paperwork at the American embassy there. We stayed overnight once again at Ruth's house in the capital city and headed back to the orphanage the next day. Every moment on this trek with Ferdie was an opportunity to become better acquainted with him and to build trust and relationship in this new family unit. Unfortunately, it was also a time for second-guessing and worrying—especially for Mary.

One of Mary's biggest fears during this time was that Ferdie was disappointed in us and, now that he was getting to know us, really didn't want to be in our family after all. There were plenty of other concerns, as well. Mary worried that Joe and Stephen, who had always been buddies in adventure, would no longer be close as another brother would now be vying for the attention of each of them. She worried that Joe and Ferdie, who both had very strong personalities, would butt heads and end up hating each other. She also worried that the special relationship she'd always had with Stephen, the "baby" of the family, would be irreparably damaged by the fact that someone else was now in that position. Mary was also troubled by her inability to say "no" to Ferdie when it was appropriate (although she'd never had any trouble doing so for her other children) and about how the extreme change to the family structure would affect the lives of each of us once back home. Despite the fact that she was completely overwhelmed with the reality she now faced and not wanting to inadvertently do or say anything that could jeopardize the false peace that she had been working so hard to portray, she tried to put on a happy face and act as if all was well. "God, please help my hurting heart!" she prayed again and again. It was her only comfort.

On the evening of the last day we were to be at the orphanage—before heading back to Ouagadougou and then home—everyone at the orphanage gathered to give Ferdie a going-away party. There were huge bowls of fish and rice, along with music, laughter, hugs, and photos. It was easy to see that Ferdie loved and was loved by so many.

The next morning, we packed the SUV, and we each took a seat in the vehicle. It was hard not to keep at least one eye on Ferdie almost constantly during this time because I was curious to see if I could determine how he was feeling. I guess I expected him to show at least a small amount of melancholy about the situation. Each time I glanced at him, though, all I could sense from him was a sense of indifference. I thought I'd see him take a few last looks around the place, stop by to give a final hug to some of his good friends, or shed a tear or two. Even as Ruth took her place behind the wheel, however, Ferdie showed no signs that he was reluctant at all about leaving. I didn't want him to have regrets about not having said a proper "goodbye" to his home, so I asked him, with Ruth's help, if he would like to do any of those things. He quickly and nonchalantly responded that he was feeling fine and that he was ready to go. So Ruth started the motor, turned the vehicle toward the gate, and eventually took us out of the courtyard onto the quiet streets of Yako for the first leg of our journey home.

We arrived in Ouagadougou a few hours before our flight was scheduled to leave, so Ruth drove us around the city and suggested a restaurant where we could get a bite to eat. As we sat at the table outside, enjoying the mild evening, Mary and I studied our surroundings carefully, knowing it would likely be quite some time before we might return to this country. Mary and the kids finished their meals with a scoop of ice cream, which was one of Ferdie's first—but certainly not his last!

When we arrived at the airport, we each grabbed our bags and began to cross the dusty ground toward the terminal. Suddenly it dawned on me that this was really, really the end of our time with Ruth and our visit to this amazing land. Funny—I knew it was coming. Still, as the security guards and gates came into view, the ending now seemed so sudden and sharp. As I turned to Ruth to say goodbye, it felt like such an inadequate gesture. How does a person, a family, thank another for all that has been done in a situation of such magnitude? It was impossible to do the situation justice, so we simply thanked her as warmly as we could and then stood back as she and Ferdie gave each other a big, final hug goodbye. Ruth uttered a few words and friendly admonitions in French to Ferdie, to which he nodded and hugged her again. What a feeling of relief and heartache it must have been for her. As she released him, she smiled once again. I put my arm around Ferdie, and together we turned and walked toward the terminal.

We were heading home with our new son.

When we boarded the plane, Ferdie was clearly nervous, but he played it pretty cool. He chose to sit next to Joe for the first half of the flight and then changed with Mary to sit next to me mid-way through. We struggled to communicate, so we didn't talk much, and he was pretty interested in the movies available to watch on the screen in front of him anyway. At one point, the movie Ferdie had chosen to watch seemed too violent to be appropriate for a child his age, but when I tried to explain that I wanted him to turn it off and choose another because of the content, I could find neither the words nor the gestures needed to explain myself to him. It was definitely a frustrating situation for both of us. In addition to the fact that Ferdie didn't fully understand the reasoning behind my decision, he also was rather unfamiliar with directives like this from someone who was supposed to be a father figure—but, in this case, was just a guy he'd met only a few days before. Standing my ground was uncomfortable, but I knew I had to do it. I tried to show him that my decision came from a place of love, but either he didn't understand or, at that point in time, it didn't really matter.

Looking back, I wonder if the situation was really about much more than the movie. Ferdie must have had an awful lot of intense emotions bouncing around inside of him at that time. I know I would have. When I consider how well he took to that experience—and many other experiences during that period in his life— I am simply in awe of his courage.

When we finally arrived home, Mary's family met us at the airport and drove home with us. They also brought us supper and served us when we got to our house. Knowing how pizza is typically a teenager's favorite meal, they presented it with a bit of a flourish, and most of us were thrilled. Ferdie, on the other hand, was less so. Like so many other things for Ferdie, pizza would take a little getting used to!

After a few days at home, Mary contacted the school to let them know Ferdie was ready to attend. Naively, we'd assumed he would be able to start the next day and were a little disappointed to hear they wanted him to wait a week or two so they could better accommodate him. Despite the fact that Ferdie left off at the fourth-grade level in Yako, he would be starting at the middle school, which contained students in grades six through eight. He was a year older than most fourth graders, so it would be more age-appropriate for him to be with the fifth-grade class. The level of support, however, would be greater at the middle school, and the school officials were adamant it was the best place for him. Mary and I weren't so sure and were a little irritated that their opinion superseded our desire for him to be with mates his age. It wasn't a battle either of us felt strongly enough to fight, though, so we agreed to take him to the middle school for his first experience with American education. Thankfully, this was the best thing that could have happened.

Ferdie was able to work in a self-contained classroom with a certified ELL (English Language Learner) instructor who assessed his level of knowledge, addressed his needs, and began to acclimate him to the American culture. She was an incredible advocate for Ferdie and quickly gained our complete confidence. Our son finished out the year working primarily with her and even continued working with her throughout the summer. By the time fall came around again, he was ready to begin his first full year of middle school at the seventh-grade level.

A few months after returning home, I thought about our adoption process. A boy who was born thousands of miles away that didn't share our genes now shared our hearts as a member of our family unit. It reminded me of how our Heavenly Father had taken all of the people from all the lands of Earth—from the past, present, and future—and welcomed everyone into *His* family. What a blessing to follow His example of faith, hope, and love.

Chapter 25

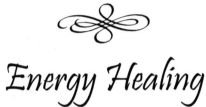

Energy Healing

Is anyone among you sick? Then he must call for the elders of the church and they are to pray over him, anointing him with oil in the name of the Lord; and the prayer of faith will restore the one who is sick, and the Lord will raise him up, and if he has committed sins, they will be forgiven him.
James 5:14-15

Even after several months, I still marveled that we finally had the family God had planned for us. Before Mary had shown me the picture of Ferdie, I couldn't in my wildest dreams have imagined I'd travel to an African country to adopt a child and love every minute of it. As Ferdie settled in and grew accustomed to life in his new family, we all settled into a new normal as well. Well, some things remained the old normal.

Maybe it was the trip to Yako or the change to our family, or maybe it was just time, but I began to feel unsettled about the progress (or lack of it) I seemed to be making with my current treatment for the chronic Lyme disease. The multiple antibiotics I'd been taking for nearly four years had helped in some ways, but it had been such a lengthy process with only minimal success. Also, in the back of my mind, I was always very aware of warnings from outside sources about the danger of antibiotic overuse, especially in the high doses I was taking. Considering the fragile condition of my stomach, I wondered if they were beginning to harm more than help me. The bottom line was I was ready for a different approach.

Around this time, I began to learn more about treatment options outside the realm of traditional Western medicine, and I couldn't help but wonder if God might be sending me signs about alternative forms of healing. One day at work, for example, a few of Mary's co-workers began talking about the use of essential oils to prevent common winter ailments such as the flu. One of the oils was said to contain compounds used hundreds of years ago to prevent individuals from contracting the Bubonic Plague. If essential oils could be effective against that bacteria, maybe it could help my body deal with the bacteria causing Lyme disease. So we purchased a diffuser, which was the suggested form of delivery, added a few drops of the recommended Thieves Oil to a small amount of water in its reservoir, and diffused it in our bedroom overnight.

When I woke up the next morning, my head was completely clear, and my breathing was strong, unlike the shallow breathing and foggy head that usually greeted me in the morning. *What a pleasant surprise!* We continued to diffuse Thieves Oil every night and consistently found the same results. Buoyed by this success, Mary and I began to consider additional oils that could be beneficial for me. One Saturday morning, Mary took out her computer and began to search for ideas. To our surprise, one of the first results led Mary to a webpage created by a woman who claimed she had been cured of chronic Lyme disease through the use of essential oils. She believed so strongly in them, in fact, that she'd created the site just to share her story with others. We were thrilled to find the website, which gave her phone number, email address, and city—which was only an hour from our home. Was this another sign from God?

The woman who responded to our email query was Pam. In her response, which occurred less than twenty-four hours after Mary sent the first message, Pam briefly described her condition, asked a bit about mine, and then offered to meet with us the following weekend. We were thrilled! For the first time in years, we felt hopeful that we might actually be able to find an effective treatment for my condition. Of course, we both had experienced too many ups and downs in the past to raise our hopes too high, but this was something new. As a result, we both experienced a level of hope we hadn't felt in a long time.

The following Saturday, after a relatively short drive, we were welcomed into Pam's home. Our conversation began with her detailing how Lyme disease had slowly and insidiously crept into her life. I found myself frequently nodding in agreement about how my hopes had been derailed so many times during this discouraging journey. Pam told us her condition had eventually even caused her to be bedridden with extreme pain, dizziness, and nausea. In her quest for healing, she'd visited numerous specialists all over the country, ringing up over $100,000 in medical expenses. As in my case, she was told by most that her symptoms could only be imaginary because the tests used by the doctors didn't reveal results beyond the boundaries of what was considered normal.

As Pam shared her story, one thing stood out: she spoke often and lovingly of her relationship with God. Time and time again, her words revealed a deep connection with Him and an immense desire to please Him. She explained she'd always known of God's presence, visualizing herself on His lap in His loving arms—a vision that I, too, had experienced. In our conversation, she revealed that her faith in God grew deeper and stronger even as her physical condition worsened. I was surprised to hear this—not because it was unbelievable to me, but rather the opposite—because I'd felt the same way myself. I guess when you're really challenged, you either run *to* God or away from Him, and we had both run to Him. It was such a comfort to honor His place in my life and to find someone here on Earth who understood it as I did.

One of the keys to Pam's healing was a natural antibiotic she used—a mixture of essential oils she called "The Magic Bullet." Pam simply put a few drops of each type, along with carrier oil, into a capsule and swallowed it. Although many people cautioned against ingesting essential oils, she asserted that it had been beneficial for her in this situation and suggested the same concoction for me. She carefully outlined the specific protocol, suggested how and where to purchase the highest quality oils, and assured me that she would guide me through the process, providing advice and support however it may be needed.

A second thing Pam suggested for me was the use of an interesting tool she had purchased called a Zyto Compass. The Zyto Compass was a machine designed to measure one's electrical impulses, and it worked simply by having the individual place their hand upon the sensor for a few minutes. Once the impulses were recorded, the machine revealed a list of nutritional supplements that would be beneficial to me. She offered me the use of her Zyto Compass as often as I'd like and once again added that she would help me obtain the suggested products.

A third suggestion from Pam was Raindrop Therapy, which Pam was certified to perform. Raindrop Therapy was an hour-long procedure in which a series of drops of multiple essential oils would be applied on the soles of my feet and along my spine. The essential oils were meant to stimulate the cells in my body to eliminate harmful bacteria and viruses, including the Lyme bacteria my body was fighting so hard to get rid of. After making an appointment with Pam for my first Raindrop Therapy, Mary and I left her house with our heads full of new knowledge and our hearts full of renewed hope.

The following week, I drove back to Pam's house for my first Raindrop Therapy. Pam and I talked for two hours before she began, and as she spoke, I again understood her story as she recognized mine—even more than the mere words used to express them. The time I spent with her that evening revealed that she was undoubtedly living out her true calling. Not one of the doctors, nurses, or other caregivers, from whom I had sought help during my many years of distress had shown the true compassion I'd found with Pam. The best part was it was all being done in God's name.

The Raindrop Therapy was very interesting itself. As I settled into place face down on her massage table, Pam began to pray. She asked God for guidance, thanked Him for His presence, and called on Him to bring healing through her hands. This act alone moved me and put me at ease. She then slowly began the process of layering the essential oils upon my body: first on my feet and then along my spine. She rubbed the oils lightly into my skin using wispy brush strokes with her hands, moving outward from my spine to each side. The process was so relaxing I was soon asleep, waking only when she placed a warm, moist towel across my shoulders, signaling the end of the therapy. I had to admit I felt refreshed, even just from the sleep.

Before I left, Pam suggested I repeat the Raindrop Therapy every ten to fourteen days. So the following Saturday, I returned for an appointment that was much the same as the first, starting with an encouraging conversation upon my arrival, then forty-five minutes of therapy. This time, however, the pain in my back, which had worsened because of my face-down position for the therapy, was increasingly hard to take. I was so glad to be there, though, and have the chance to talk to someone with whom I had so much in common and who'd overcome something I wanted so much to beat myself that I didn't say anything. The hope I was feeling about the treatment was like a breath of fresh air to someone who'd been forced to breathe only heavy, stale air for far too long.

In the middle of my next Rainbow Therapy session, however, when the discomfort in my back returned, I decided to mention it to Pam. She responded by asking if she could do something a little different that day, to which I agreed. She applied the oil as she'd done several times before, then left for a bit. When she returned, she asked where it hurt, then laid her hands on that spot. For the next few minutes, I heard her speaking softly to herself but couldn't make out what she was saying. Afterward, she spoke a little louder, clearly addressing me.

Pam told me that she believed that my back was aching because cells in that area were imbalanced as a result of a sickness I'd had when I was four years old and a very emotional experience I'd had with a former girlfriend when I was seventeen years old. I was shocked by her revelation. First, because I immediately recognized the situations to which she referred. Second, because it amazed me that she had been able to recognize them with such specificity, without any input on my part, right down to the age that I'd been at the times of those events—or almost, anyway, since she was right regarding my age for the incident with my girlfriend and only a year off about the situation that had occurred in my childhood. How was she able to do that? What did she mean about my cells being imbalanced? It all sounded very strange.

Although Pam's words astounded and confused me, I'd developed a strong bond with her over the past month or so and completely trusted her actions and intentions. As she continued applying the essential oils to my body, I thought about what she'd said. So far from falling asleep this time, I could hardly wait for her to finish the procedure so I could ask her to explain what she had meant when she referred to my cells being "unbalanced by my emotions." Since I didn't yet notice any major change in my backache, I, of course, wondered if what she had said could really be true and if what she had done could possibly help.

When Pam had finished my therapy, I slowly arose from the table, regained my bearings, then made my way to the nearby couch while she put things away and tidied the area. I tried to gauge whether or not what she had done for my back had helped or if I might just be imagining it did—or didn't. I wasn't sure but hoped I would have a better idea about it as time went on. Pam joined me in the sitting area a few minutes later, and I eagerly asked her to tell me more about what she had done.

Pam began by explaining that everything is made of energy, and our bodies are no different. Even things like thoughts and feelings are made of energy. As our physical bodies move through life, they are affected by the energies around them. Some of the energies pass through our cells without effect, while others affect them for the better or have a negative effect.

When a person experiences emotions that are not processed appropriately by the individual, they have a negative effect on one's cells, causing the cells to vibrate in unnatural ways. The vibrations are imperceptible to the person overall, but on a cellular level, the distortion is very real, and its effect can be huge. Unbalanced cells lead to an unbalanced body which results in physical discomfort, among other things. The concept, she elaborated, was based on the teachings of Doctor Bradley Nelson and was known as The Body Code.

The Body Code, Pam explained, is a method of interacting with the body by asking it yes or no questions, then listening for the body's response. The body's response is measured through muscle testing. A person's muscles temporarily weaken to indicate a "false" or "no" response and maintain strength for a "positive" or "yes" response.

Pam was probably somewhat ready for my incredulity about what she had done and the continuous line of questioning that followed, so she took considerable time to explain the principles of The Body Code for an hour or more until I finally felt like I understood what she was saying, even if I wasn't sure yet what I believed about everything she said. When she had finished, I reiterated how amazed I was at what I had learned and thanked her for taking so much time to help me comprehend such new and usual ideas. Before I left, though, I wanted to clarify something she'd said. It wasn't a big deal at the time, but I wanted to give her the chance to consider what she'd told me to bolster her credibility regarding The Body Code.

I wanted to give Pam another chance to think about what she'd told me while she was helping relieve my back pain during the Raindrop Therapy. Something she'd said wasn't exactly right, and I didn't want to leave without addressing it. While somehow, Pam had accurately identified my age in the situation where my girlfriend had broken up with me in high school (the situation she claimed was causing my back discomfort), she was close but not quite right in her estimate of my age when I'd become so sick in my youth. I had, after all, always known I was five years old during that incident—not four, as she'd said. When I brought this up, her response surprised me. She told me there was a chance of her exaggerating the time by a year, but in this case, she was pretty sure I really was four years old when I'd been sick. I didn't feel the need to argue the point, but I knew she was wrong. The fact that she'd been anywhere close to identifying my age during two traumatic periods in my life was quite amazing, even if she wasn't spot-on for both of them. It's safe to say that I left Pam's house that day a bit skeptical but certainly intrigued.

On my way home, I tried once again to analyze whether or not my back was feeling better, but I still wasn't sure. There was one thing I did know, though: Pam's ability to recognize those significant life issues she'd uncovered during that day's session was incredible. I thought about it all the way home. It didn't stop upon my arrival there, however, as it was the first thing out of my mouth in my conversation with Mary as soon as I got home and still remained foremost in my thoughts throughout the week and into the weekend. That Sunday, when I visited my mom, I took the opportunity to ask her how old I had been when I was sick. "Why, you were just four," she told me confidently.

"What? I wasn't five?" I asked.

"No, you were definitely four," she confirmed.

Wow. This was definitely unexpected news, and it was a little eerie, to say the least.

Although I didn't realize it until later, Pam's use of energy healing wasn't my first experience with this unusual concept. A few years before, I was having physical reactions to most foods, so there wasn't much, if anything, I could safely eat without having some kind of side effect. I had already lost quite a bit of weight and was ready to grab onto anything I could that might be helpful. My niece was the receptionist at a nearby chiropractor's office. The chiropractor, she told me, had a unique approach to reducing allergic reactions. My niece's husband had, in fact, already tried it in an attempt to lessen his seasonal allergies and felt that it had been effective. Always in search of help of almost any kind, I'd jumped at the opportunity.

When I arrived at the chiropractor on the day of my visit, I was shown to a small room with a cot. I waited only a few minutes before the chiropractor opened the door, greeted me, and sat beside me at his desk. After a bit of small talk, he asked me about my specific health concerns. I told him about my numerous food intolerances/allergies, including a bit about how it was probably quicker and easier to tell him what things I didn't have a problem with than the many that I did. He listened intently as I spoke and, when I'd finished, stood up and began to look through a collection of vials on a nearby shelf. Eventually, he selected one, put the entire vial in a small jar, and returned to his desk.

The chiropractor then asked me to lie face down on the cot. Once I had situated myself there, he handed me the jar containing the vial and began to adjust my body as he would for a typical chiropractic appointment. While he worked, he began to tell me about the procedure. The treatment, he said, was based on the work done by a chiropractor in California named Devi Nambudripad. It was referred to as NAET (Nambudripad's Allergy Elimination Technique) and was a form of applied kinesiology. To be honest, I didn't follow much of what he was saying at the time because I was still rather preoccupied with the notion that holding a little vial inside of another glass container could do anything to affect how I felt or how my body reacted to the world around me. It wasn't like I was doubting it because I wasn't, but it was just such a foreign concept. Nonetheless, if it helped, I didn't much care how realistic or crazy it sounded; I just wanted relief!

After about ten minutes, the chiropractor told me he was finished and suggested that I come back for several more appointments in the coming weeks. Definitely. If this helped, I'd come back as often as I could!

While I spoke with my niece, the receptionist, to make my next appointment, I slowly began to notice that my chest and upper arms were starting to itch. She recognized it in me almost before I could mention it myself and immediately highlighted that many people have a similar response after a session. She told me not to worry, though, because the discomfort was typically mild and short-lived. I wouldn't have characterized the physical response I was having in that way, but in the end, the situation never became serious and eventually did go away without any significant reason to worry.

I continued to visit this chiropractor once a week throughout the winter. Each time, he gave me a different vial to hold, and most of the time, I had a similar reaction that typically subsided by the time I arrived home an hour later. By the time spring arrived, I'd completed treatment with all of the vials. Unfortunately, I was still having a lot of trouble finding foods to eat that didn't seem to affect my body or mind negatively. Consequently, I didn't know whether or not his treatments were beneficial, and throughout the following summer months, I was still not certain anything had changed.

When ragweed season arrived in the fall, though, my body's tolerance for the pollen was noticeably improved. I sneezed less, my eyes didn't water as much, and my body seemed less sensitive to foods that typically seemed to cause a negative reaction in my body and mind. In the end, even though NAET treatment was not the cure-all I was seeking, the fact that it was able to help me better cope with my yearly ragweed allergies was definitely a blessing. Who knows, perhaps the NAET was subtly working in other ways to provide the relief my body would need to heal. I'll likely never know for sure—not while here on Earth, anyway.

Now, back to the present. Was the NAET energy work done by the chiropractor years ago related somehow to what Pam was doing, or was it something entirely different? Even more important, was it a method for healing that was in alignment with God's teaching? It was definitely unusual, but did that automatically mean it was something God would forbid?

Leviticus 19:31 tells us, "Do not turn to mediums or spiritists; do not seek them out to be defiled by them. I am the LORD your God." It is also written, however, in James 5:14, "Is anyone among you sick? *Then* he must call for the elders of the church and they are to pray over him, anointing him with oil in the name of the Lord."

Wasn't this, in essence, what Pam was doing? Could I consider her an elder of the church who was praying over me, anointing me with oil in the name of God? If not—if what she was doing was against God's teachings—I'd rather be sick.

Chapter 26

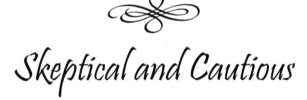

Skeptical and Cautious

*Do not turn to mediums or spiritists; do
not seek them out to be defiled by them.
I am the LORD your God.*
Leviticus 19:31

When my mom confirmed the date of my childhood illness, my incredulity about Pam's ability to recognize something within me that I hadn't even seen myself increased, and my mind swirled with questions well before I approached Pam's home for my next appointment. I'd spent a lot of time wondering about the legitimacy of her treatment, but most of all, questioning whether or not what she was doing would be offensive to God. I didn't want to sin, even if doing so might take away my physical pain.

I'd been looking for a sign from God to help me decide whether or not I should proceed with Pam's radically different form of healing. As usual, God didn't speak to me in the clear, loud voice that would have made it so easy. So I tried to determine His wishes by searching His Word in the Bible, praying to Him, listening for Him, and looking for other clues wherever they may be.

The Bible says in Deuteronomy 18: 9-12:

When you enter the land which the Lord your God is giving you,

you shall not learn to imitate the detestable things of those nations. There shall not be found among you anyone who makes his son or his daughter pass through the fire, one who uses divination, a soothsayer, one who interprets omens, or a sorcerer, or one who casts a spell, or a medium, or a spiritist, or one who consults the dead. For whoever does these things is detestable to the Lord; and because of these detestable things the Lord your God is going to drive them out before you.

Pam didn't do any of those things.

Similarly, Leviticus 20:6 says, "As for the person who turns to mediums and to spiritists, to play the prostitute with them, I will also set My face against that person and will cut him off from among his people." Pam wasn't a medium or a spiritist, either.

Nothing I found in the Bible appeared to condemn what Pam was doing. Still, since I was confused about whether or not this was a course of action I should follow, I began to pray even more intensely for God to just show me how to obey Him. I prayed that, above all, He would guide me to do the right thing and asked Him to close this door of opportunity if it was something I shouldn't be doing.

In addition to talking to God about this form of healing, I also talked to Pam. I trusted her opinion because I knew how intensely she loved God. We talked for many hours about the situation. She always listened patiently and responded thoughtfully to every question and concern.

In the end, I came to a conclusion that felt right in my heart and my head. Since I'd found nothing in the Word that seemed to forbid Pam's actions, I decided to proceed with her treatment. I was further reassured by Pam's prayers for guidance before each session and the fact that she gave God glory for every bit of healing that occurred afterward. I was also further comforted that she never sought information about the future, which we both knew God clearly prohibited.

Once I'd come to terms with the question about whether or not God would approve of this form of healing, my thoughts next landed upon the idea of whether or not these techniques would actually, truly heal me. Obviously, neither Mary nor I wanted to spend a lot of time or money on something that wouldn't yield positive results, as we'd done so many times before. Even so, we were encouraged that this alternative method addressed the healing of my whole self (even my spiritual) rather than just the physical symptoms of disease. Maybe this was critical to my healing. Also, we were drawn to Pam's compassion, which was so different from what treatment I'd experienced before. It was hard not to be influenced by her genuine willingness to help.

While I considered the treatment that Pam offered, I remembered my experiences with the chiropractor who'd used the NAET protocol with me. His treatment hadn't diminished my food intolerances (a claim I'd hoped for, though it wasn't one he'd ever made), but it did significantly diminish my ragweed allergies, which was such a blessing. Perhaps the same would happen with Pam. Maybe her treatment wouldn't eliminate everything that ailed me, but it would at least lessen the severity or remove some components of the problem. At this point, the option of feeling even a little better was enticing.

For several months, Pam continued to focus on the unprocessed negative emotions affecting my cells. While I had experienced some of the negative emotions within the past five or ten years, Pam believed what was affecting my health had occurred when I was a very young child. She even went so far as to suggest some of them had been experienced while in utero—had been passed to me genetically through my parents or ancestors well before I was born. I'm not going to pretend that some of what she told me didn't blow my mind. In fact, Mary and I had many conversations during which we both agreed that we weren't sure if what was being said to us was true or just an obscure claim.

With help from Google, Mary discovered that Pam's healing method was called *energy psychology* (EP). According to Google sources, Mary learned that EP is based on quantum physics and spirituality. Quantum physics theorizes that since all matter is made of energy, the particles of energy in any type of material (physical objects such as furniture and elements of nature such as body cells, etc.) and even non-material things (intangible items such as thoughts, feelings, etc.) affect and are affected by each other.

Energy psychology is similar to traditional psychology in that it strives to positively affect physical and mental health through discussion and relationship building. Energy psychology has many variations. One of them is Nambudripad's Allergy Elimination Techniques (NAET), which I'd already experienced many times with the chiropractor who'd asked me to hold vials of different environmental allergens while he adjusted my body. Other variations include the Emotional Freedom Technique (EFT), Energy Consciousness Therapy (ECT), and Doctor Bradley Nelson's Emotion Code and Body Code methods.

Pam used the latter of these options: Doctor Nelson's Emotion and Body Codes. Doctor Nelson's method proposes that unprocessed past emotions are trapped in the body's cells, causing them to vibrate unnaturally, which results in stress, pain, and disease. A series of questions enables the practitioner to identify the cause of the trapped emotions and release them, thereby returning the cell to healthy functioning. A body potentially has thousands of trapped emotions, so the release of one or two may or may not be the lynchpin needed for recognizable healing. Furthermore, it may take many, many more releases to find the one exact cell whose rebalance will affect enough of the cells to relieve one's discomfort.

One of Pam's first efforts was to try to eliminate the unhealthy emotions that were causing unnatural vibrations in the cells surrounding my heart. She told me that when negative emotions are trapped in that region, it is called a "heart wall." The subconscious mind creates a heart wall in an attempt to shield oneself from pain. Although a heart wall sounds like it would be a good thing, it isn't good because the unnatural vibrations of the cell result in pain and discomfort, preventing one from experiencing positive emotions and makes it difficult for individuals to form emotional connections with others.

When Pam first began to work on my heart wall, she told me it was the equivalent of seventy-five miles thick and was as hard as steel. After the first session, she was able to decrease it slightly, but it took several more sessions to reduce it to nearly half its original thickness. In addition to treating my heart wall, Pam treated other cells throughout my body, releasing emotions such as abandonment, terror, overwhelm and despair, and a lot of emotions she labeled "willingness to die."

As unusual as it seemed at the time, I was less critical of Pam's unusual methods than I ever would have been before. I wanted so much to be relieved of my discomfort that I was willing to try anything, within the realm of what God would allow, anyway. I was hoping and praying that perhaps Pam's techniques would identify and remove the root of whatever was ailing me in ways that traditional medicine had not yet been able to accomplish.

In addition to using Doctor Nelson's Body and Emotion Code methods, Pam also strongly believed in using essential oils. She had a vast knowledge of them and a thick reference book always close at hand when she had a question. To determine which essential oil to use, she simply asked me about my symptoms, took a few moments to consider an essential oil that might be helpful, and then held a vial of that oil in her hands while muscle testing to determine if it would or wouldn't be beneficial to me. If the response indicated that it was a good choice, she would ask how it should be used (rubbed on, misted in the air, or taken orally), how much should be used, and how often it should be used, relying once again on muscle testing to identify the correct response. Sometimes she invited me to use her Zyto Compass, a device that matched deficiencies in the electrical impulses in my hand to the frequency of a wide variety of essential oils and other supplements.

As my exposure to essential oils grew, Mary began to investigate them to learn more about what they were and how they worked. She discovered that essential oils are strong concentrations acquired from plants through a distillation process. The molecules of essential oils are tiny, making it easy for them to permeate the cells. Essential oils carry terpenes that are believed to release toxins being held in the body and inhibit new ones from forming. The molecules also carry other benefits: esters, anti-bacterial, anti-inflammatory, anti-fungal, and antiviral ketones that promote cell regeneration; oxides that are antiseptics and expectorants; alcohols that invigorate the immune system; and phenols that provide fragrance and aldehydes that are calming when inhaled. While traditional medicine doesn't support the use of essential oils, there are numerous success stories from people otherwise unable to find relief that tout their effectiveness.

The information we found sounded promising, but I'd heard a lot of promising things before that which hadn't, in the end, amounted to much. The problem I now faced was that I was basically at a dead end with traditional Western medicine and still felt miserable, so I needed to do something. Long, unsuccessful years of seeking relief from doctors in clinics and hospitals from all over had opened my mind to new ideas and possibilities. I'd come to the conclusion that I'd try just about anything as long as it didn't go against one key principle: God's Word. After further contemplation, then, it seemed both logical and biblically acceptable to use treatments derived from the plants God had put on Earth, which is what the use of essential oils appeared to do. Thus, I continued to welcome Pam's advice and invested myself in using essential oils as she saw fit. I also continued to be open to other alternative methods God may have for my health.

It was at this point in my life—after having met Pam and hearing about her struggles and triumphs and the stories of others who had found relief from ailments outside of traditional medicine—that I began to sense a call from God to write about my life. I didn't know who He wanted me to write it for or exactly what He wanted me to say. I just began to feel He wanted me to write my story. For someone who struggles so much with reading and writing, the idea that I would undertake such a large writing project seemed rather ridiculous. It certainly wasn't in my comfort zone, nor something I considered fun to do. Nevertheless, God kept after me until I eventually just put a pencil to paper and simply began to write.

At about this same time, Pam made the decision to stop using Doctor Bradley Nelson's Body Code method to help release trapped emotions. She continued to provide Raindrop Therapy and Emotion Code services but chose to stop administering The Body Code treatment—for the time being, at least. When I asked her about her decision, she told me that she'd been feeling uncomfortable about how she'd undergone the process of learning this more thorough (and more expensive) type of treatment. The issue, she said, was that she'd borrowed the pricey videotape set and manuals from an acquaintance but had never actually purchased them herself. She'd sensed God communicating with her about this, telling her that it wasn't an honest way to do business. Unfortunately, Pam couldn't currently afford to purchase the materials on her own. Therefore, until she could, she would no longer use those techniques.

Since Pam no longer offered healing through The Body Code, my options for treatment were now much more limited and certainly made me pause and think about whether or not I should continue to work with her. I tried to analyze how much she'd helped me but eventually came to the conclusion that, although I was feeling better, I had no measurable evidence to explain why or how. I recognized that my anxiety had decreased throughout the past few months and that I was more consciously and, therefore, more positively reacting to negative situations in my life than I'd done previously. Still, these were rather intangible concepts, and although they were very welcomed, the level of improvement was rather hard to determine, which made any type of decision difficult.

After considerable time and prayer, I decided that since Pam was no longer able to provide The Body Code treatment, it would be best for me to find someone else who could. As you might imagine, this was a very bittersweet decision for me. I was so inspired by Pam's devotion and loved having her pray over and for me. It would be extremely difficult to replace that kind of care and the depth in which I was immersed in God's love during her treatments.

During the following months, I continued to see Pam occasionally for Raindrop Therapy and checked in with her once in a while to see how she was doing. Meanwhile, Mary and I turned our attention to another healer we had found who would be able to provide further treatment for me at an even more convenient location—my own home.

At that time, Doctor Bradley Nelson's webpage had a map displaying the location and contact information of trained Body and Emotion Code providers around the world. Mary and I were pleasantly surprised to discover there was more than one of them in Wisconsin. So one day, after asking God for guidance, Mary clicked the dot on the map that led us to a woman named Renee, who would become the next link in my chain of healers.

Renee had trained directly under Doctor Nelson. She had been practicing energy healing for years. In addition, she'd been exposed to a number of holistic healing methods as a child, so her appreciation for unique treatments had developed early in her life. She'd previously been an accountant, working with information that was measurable and exact. Over time, however, her innate gift of intuition became difficult to ignore, and she eventually found herself moving away from facts and figures toward a career permeated by feelings and beliefs.

Renee did much of her energy work via the telephone. Her appointments were forty-five minutes long, give or take fifteen minutes of conversation before, during, and after the actual session. She'd begin by calling me on the phone, and then, as with Pam, she worked on eliminating negative issues. Over time, many of my symptoms lessened, and once again, I became hopeful that I would eventually find complete healing. Unfortunately, despite numerous sessions with Renee and her release of countless negative emotions, nothing that was eliminated seemed to be the lynchpin that resolved whatever it was that kept me so unwell.

As had occurred so many times before, one particular symptom again eventually rose to the top of my list of discomforts. This time it was my back. It was an old ache, actually, one I'd felt since I was about eighteen years old. It came and went with varying degrees of distress—sometimes barely noticeable and others so intense I could hardly get out of bed. I'd tried heating pads, ice packs, bathtub soaks, back massages, chiropractors, essential oils, and magnetic therapy. Of course, once I found them, I'd had Pam and Renee both address the issue, as well. It would have been less of an issue if my body could have tolerated ibuprofen, acetaminophen, or medical salves, but the use of any of those types of things just led to additional negative issues.

Despite the pain I was experiencing, I probably would have stuck to my earlier promise of staying away from traditional Western medicine, but at one point I began to notice an increase in the amount of blood in my stool and urine. For years blood had been evident there, so this wasn't new. I'd done cancer screenings several times in the past to ensure that the blood wasn't a symptom of anything serious. Since the tests had always come back negative, the doctors concluded that the blood was probably related to constipation and/or the ulcerative colitis in my system.

This time, though, the volume and frequency of the blood had increased as the back pain intensified, and the symptoms didn't let up as they had in the past. Still, I'd been through this so many times before: "This is serious. I'd better get to a doctor!" crisis had always turned out to be a big Nothing Burger—with a Big Something-Burger medical bill attached to it. So I tried everything one more time, including the wait-it-out method. Unfortunately, as weeks and months passed, and the situation didn't improve, my discomfort and the concern it could really be something serious this time became stronger than my patience. So one afternoon after work, I went to see the physician's assistant to find out what he could suggest.

I had no idea this would lead me to yet another venture into alternative medicine, which in turn would completely clarify the direction I should take—and just might lead to the remedy I had been searching for all my life.

Chapter 27

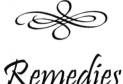

Remedies

*Every moving thing that is alive shall be food
for you; I have given everything to you,
as I gave the green plant.*
Genesis 9:3

When the physician's assistant called me less than twelve hours later, I knew what he had to say couldn't be good. He told me the lab results showed blood in my urine, and it was critical I see a urologist immediately to determine the cause of the bleeding. He couldn't say if my back problems were related, but if it wasn't, treatment could be pursued afterward.

I was two weeks shy of an appointment with a highly regarded local homeopath. I'd scheduled it almost two years earlier, but the homeopath's schedule was so full that I'd had to wait eighteen months to see her. A few acquaintances had told me that this specialist would be able to provide information and remedies not available from anyone else. Since the appointment was just a few days away, I seriously considered ignoring the phone call and just waiting for the homeopath to deal with the situation. After all, I'd had plenty of reasons by then to assume that traditional medicine wouldn't be beneficial for me, anyway.

Although my plan made sense at the time, things changed within just a few days when searing pain drove me to seek immediate relief, which was only available through an appointment with a urologist. When I was able to make an appointment within just a few days, I was pleasantly surprised and was immediately hopeful that this was a sign from God that I'd made the right decision. Regardless, I was in a whole lot of pain, so both Mary and I were nervous that whatever was going on was pretty serious.

During our drive to the clinic on the day of my appointment, our minds seemed fixated on two potential discoveries. One, that the pain in my back was caused by something that was ultimately responsible for all the physical troubles I'd been plagued with throughout my life. Now that it was discovered, both my back pain and my overall health would finally be restored. Two, that the condition was caused by cancer and my time here on Earth would soon be over. Needless to say, Mary and I were both a little tense. After parking the car, we remained there for a few moments to pray for strength, wisdom for the doctor, and of course, my healing—one way or another.

The receptionist at the clinic greeted us with a warm smile and chatted pleasantly, obviously unaware of the life-and-death nature of the appointment. After she took my name and insurance card, she directed us to the waiting room, highlighting that the nurse would be with us in just a few minutes. Since we were the only ones there, we assumed she was right and were barely seated before my name was called. I was then taken back to an exam room where the nurse took my vitals, gave me a gown and a small plastic container, and directed me to a nearby restroom so I could collect a urine sample.

After my specimen had been delivered, it took a surprisingly small amount of time for the results to be reported back to me. Given my track record of having intense situations turn out to be absolutely nothing, I shouldn't have been surprised when the nurse came back to let me know that the amount of blood in the sample I'd provided was so little it could barely even be measured and was, most definitely, not at all a threat to my overall well-being. My initial sigh of relief at the news was almost immediately replaced with a sigh of resignation at yet one more instance where clarity seemed so hard to find. "Now what?" I almost growled. If this back pain wasn't because of a kidney issue or some type of cancer, what was causing it?

Although he didn't know much about other possible causes for lower back pain, the urologist suggested that an ultrasound or a CAT scan might help identify whether a hernia or disk problem could be the cause of my pain. *Boom.* Here I was, right back where I'd been just a few days ago. I was again in the position of deciding whether it was logical for me to seek help from someone in the field of Western medicine or if I would be better off pursuing support from a different kind of specialist, such as one in the field of alternative medicine. On the one hand, we'd already traveled halfway down this path with the traditional physician. Therefore, it seemed logical to continue it, especially since it now seemed likely that my back pain was the result of some type of structural issue, a condition that a traditional physician would be adept at healing. This option also offered financial support from insurance, which made the situation at least a little more enticing. On the other hand, I'd already experienced so many occasions where Western medicine seemed the obvious choice, yet in the end, it didn't help at all. To make matters worse, most of those times resulted in me just owing the hospital or clinic a considerable sum of money with absolutely no improvements to my health. My appointment with the homeopath was just around the corner, after all. Even so, since insurance companies don't provide financial support when working with a homeopath, the alternative medicine route could end up being extremely expensive, too.

My mind kept jumping from one reason to another for seeking relief from traditional or alternative specialists. For every good argument against one, there was a good argument for the opposite until I finally decided to stop thinking about it for a while and hoped that time might clarify the situation for me one way or the other.

Somewhere along the way, God pushed His way to the front of my muddled mind, and my path was finally made straight. While Western medicine works through synthetic pills and resources that are devoid of faith in God, the best health care was provided by people who love and honor Him and who use resources He placed in nature for our healing. The course of action, then, was clear; I decided to forgo any further testing at the medical clinic and simply wait for my appointment with the homeopath. Incredibly, I received a phone call only a few days later from a staff member at the office of the homeopath. The date of my appointment was right around the corner, but there had been a cancellation that presented me with the opportunity to come even a few days earlier. It was as if God was affirming my choice, showing me that I'd made the right decision this time.

Remedies is a homeopathic clinic in Oshkosh we'd heard about two years earlier from a high school classmate of mine. She couldn't say enough about how Remedies had improved her health. A classmate told me after church one day that Nicki, the specialist, was an extremely gifted homeopath. Anyone who has been sick for a long time and/or unable to find relief elsewhere knows how quickly and tightly one grabs onto hope of any kind in that department. So it was for me with Remedies. When Monday morning rolled around, I was on the phone as soon as the clinic opened to get my name in the appointment book. Imagine my astonishment when I was told that the earliest date I could be scheduled was almost two years away!

One could argue that such a long wait was actually a good thing. After all, if a specialist is in such high demand, she must really be good. Unfortunately, I wasn't that one. The plain fact of the matter was that I didn't know if I could wait that long—either mentally or physically. Honestly, there were periods of time when I truly wondered if I could make it even one more week. Somewhere deep down, though, I heard a small voice of reassurance "You've kept your faith this long, John—don't blow it now. Take this one day at a time. The date will get here eventually. You can do it!"

And I did.

On the day I finally entered Remedies, my back was full of pain, but my heart was full of hope. We arrived a few minutes early, so I took a seat in the waiting room and studied my surroundings. Most of the clinic was filled from floor to ceiling with shelves upon which supplements and personal care items had been carefully arranged. A few pleasant staff members bustled around answering the phone, working with other customers, and preparing various mailings. Then, precisely on time, a woman approached us with an outstretched hand in greeting.

The woman introduced herself as Nicki, and Mary and I immediately warmed to her smiling face. She invited us back to her office, and we enthusiastically followed, sharing a glance that said, *"This is it!"*

My first visit was a five-hour appointment. You read that right: *five* hours. I'd personally never heard of such a thing, but if it meant getting to the bottom of whatever was wrong with me, I'd have stayed all day—or longer. Nicki offered me a comfortable leather chair in the corner of the room and sat down herself at a desk upon which a large computer and screen had been placed. She began to review the paperwork I'd completed and brought along, which had been sent to me by the clinic after I'd initially made the appointment so many months ago. It contained information about my symptoms, health history, and goals for healing. I hoped I'd given her everything that was pertinent to my situation because I sure didn't want to mess anything up!

After a few niceties, Nicki got right to work. She began by explaining her view of disease by highlighting it as a body's dis-ease—or lack of comfort. For example, on the Remedies website, Nicki writes:

> Imbalances in the body are the origins of your symptomology. Our goal is to find the causes of the problems and eliminate them. Once the causes are eliminated, the body can then begin to balance and heal itself, resulting in good health in both body and mind.

In Nicki's explanation, she tried to clarify the body's response to the imbalances that lead to physical and mental discomforts, but even her simplification of the process was beyond my scope of understanding. Still, I tried to keep up with her discussion, but in the end was fine with not understanding the details and happy just to be working with someone who was sure she could bring me some relief. I wasn't as interested in the process as I was in the product—I just wanted to feel better!

Once she'd tried to help me understand why my body wasn't working properly and how she was going to fix it, Nicki handed me a brass cylinder. It was about three inches long and about an inch in diameter. It was wrapped in a wet paper towel, which she'd deftly prepared for me as she'd likely done hundreds of times over the course of her work. Nicki explained that this was a grounding bar and was necessary for me to hold in my left hand while she worked with the fingers on my right.

Once I was settled with my feet flat on the floor, the grounding bar in my left hand and my right hand outstretched toward her, Nicki began to touch specific points on my fingers using a metal stylus to begin the process of electrodermal screening. She told me that she was touching specific points on my hand called meridians and that they were energy and information pathways that ran throughout my body. Nicki explained that in doing this, the right side of my body was communicating with the left side of my brain. The left side of my brain then sent information back to my right, which she then measured with her probe. The measurement was sent via the stylus to her computer and organized there in a way that enabled her to determine the location and level of my body's imbalances, converting numerical values received through the stylus to more qualitative readings with terminology such as "healthy," "within normal limits," "subacute," or "acute." I learned the process is not very different from the core principles of electrocardiography, which uses skin surface electrical patterns to assess heart function.

The entire process seemed bizarre to me, but I wasn't skeptical. Of course, I wasn't sure how it all was supposed to work, but somehow I trusted Nicki. Each time she touched one of my fingers with the stylus, the machine made a brief humming sound, then sent a reading to the computer's screen. She then clicked a key on the computer. The same procedure was repeated for the next five hours—touch the finger with the stylus, watch the result on the screen, then click a key on the computer. Although it might seem like it should have been an excruciatingly monotonous time, it was nothing of the sort. As she worked, Nicki freely talked about her life and asked me about mine. I could tell right away she was an incredibly intelligent woman who had used her gifts to accomplish many interesting things. Most of all, we recognized she was in awe of the One who was behind everything in this world. She loved God, crediting and trusting Him above all else.

The locations where Nicki began to probe were derived from the information I'd provided on the questionnaire I'd completed. Once the frequencies in the problem areas were measured, Nicki matched them to potential homeopathic remedies with a corresponding frequency to see which one best aligned with the body. "Your body actually chooses the remedy!" Nicki highlighted. The best part, she said, was that "one supplement may take care of numerous problems or issues. Our bodies' systems are so intricately intertwined and complicated that our symptoms may be far from the actual cause."

Nicki went on to explain that products can range from therapies, homeopathics, and nutritional supplements to herbs, flower remedies, and phenolic isodes. Before recommending them, however, she would go over each product and modality by asking your body which items are safe, tolerable, beneficial, and effective. An item must be all of the above to be suggested.

Nicki then told me more about how sometimes one product alone will not balance a person. Therefore, other modalities (chiropractic adjustments, far-infrared saunas, footbaths, lymph star treatments, IVs, massage, cranial sacral treatments, acupuncture, etc.) are necessary in conjunction with other products to bring about optimal health.

The information Nicki presented was fascinating. The difference between Western medicine and Nicki's homeopathic approach was mind-blowing. How could this be? Had there been a mistake along the way somewhere by the "healing decision makers" (whoever they may be) so that one form of healing was actually wrong and the other form actually correct? Or was there a unique place and time in which one would be appropriate that the other would not? Shouldn't there be more of a public discussion somewhere about the pros and cons of each so that some type of recommendation or compromise could be reached? Why did it seem like homeopathic medicine was being performed in relative obscurity, far in the shadow cast in our country by the mighty monolith of Western medicine?

Throughout my appointment and later at home, I learned more about electrodermal screening. What I discovered was fascinating! *The meridian energy system that was the basis for Nicki's work wasn't just an interesting hypothesis—it had been scientifically observed in a peer-researched study*[3]. Electrodermal screening tests confirmed the flow of energy in pathways through internal organs and along the surface of the skin. The electrodermal screening device (i.e., Nicki's stylus) measures electrical resistance and polarization at specific points and meridians. Scientists correspond points on the skin

---

3   Chen, C.W. et al. (2013) *Wave-induced Flow in Meridians Demonstrated Using Photoluminescent Bioceramic Material on Acupuncture Points, Evidence-based Complementary and Alternative Medicine: eCAM*. U.S. National Library of Medicine. Available at: https://www.ncbi.nlm.nih.gov/pmc/articles/PMC3838801/.

to certain meridians, which they refer to as "organ projection areas." Touching an organ projection area with the electrodermal screening device enabled the energy in the corresponding organ or body system to be manipulated so it would function more effectively. It also enabled the healer to measure the energy flow in an organ or body system to diagnose imbalances in the body that could eventually lead to disease.

As Nicki ran the tests, I felt completely comfortable and extremely hopeful. Perhaps it was because she'd convinced me of the scientific legitimacy of her process and the fact that her healing techniques would include resources taken from God's creation, which is so important to me. I was also touched by Nicki's compassion, which was such a stark and welcoming contrast to the care I'd received in most clinics throughout my life.

As we approached the end of hour five and thus the conclusion of my appointment, Nicki put down the stylus, took the grounding bar from my hand, and began to print some documents from her computer. She then began to tell me about every parasite, virus, and infection I had ever experienced. She explained I had trouble digesting food because I didn't have the enzymes needed to do so and highlighted that I still had remnants of Lyme disease to clean up, along with residual co-infections of Bartonella and Babesia—and said she could help with all of it. In addition, of course, she would help relieve the pain in my back and the blood in my urine. She assured me she had a remedy for everything ailing me.

Nicki then handed me a packet of information explaining in greater detail each of her findings and a list of remedies she recommended to help my body heal from each issue. I was thrilled to see and hear that each of her suggestions was a substance derived from nature—from God. Each of them had been selected because of its ability to help my body build healthy cells and eliminate elements that were causing some type of harm.

As a bonus of sorts, Nicki concluded by telling me that whoever was doing my energy work was doing a great job because those efforts had helped my body release a significant amount of energy that was preventing my healing. This was an unexpected but welcome addition to the rest of the news I'd received from her. I felt so blessed!

As we walked out of the clinic that evening, Mary and I were sure we couldn't be in better hands—hands of love, faith, and strength. It was yet another reminder of God's providence and care. He had shown me repeatedly throughout my life that He was always with me and that He had blessed my life when I sought godly resources to meet my needs. I hadn't always noticed that, however—nor appreciated it. Looking back now, though, I recognize that God really did have a team of people waiting to help me through every step of my challenges. Most recently, those helpers included my high school friend, Vicki, who'd introduced me to Mannatech and the Ambrotose supplement. Then there was Doctor Aaron, who prayed with me before and after every session and introduced me to Doctor M., who had allowed me to work with his assistant, who'd uncovered the chronic Lyme disease diagnosis. Next was Rebecca, whose antibiotic regimen, while lovingly administered, wasn't able to eradicate the disease and thus caused me to seek healing outside the realm of traditional Western medical practices. God's path continued with Pam, who showed me the power of essential oils, energy healing, and, most of all, prayer. Soon after Pam came Renee, who continued the energy work of removing roadblocks hindering my healing that were beyond my consciousness. Finally came Nicki, the healer whose use of yet another unique technique was able to identify still more issues and provided options for healing, each one of them using resources from God's creation. What a journey it had been.

God's path for my life took me on a course I didn't enjoy and didn't understand. I like to think God knew I'd never leave Him, no matter what kind of hell I had to face, so maybe He picked me for a special challenge. Perhaps He needed someone to tell others about faith and perseverance and finding a God-way of healing. When I meet Him in Heaven, I'm certainly going to ask. Until then, knowing that He might have used me and my life of misery to lessen someone else's pain, through the avenue of this book, for example, I am truly honored. I hope I have done that for you.

Author's Note

I sat on this book for a long time, not wanting to finish it. I was hoping by the time I was all done, I would be totally healed so I could show off a miracle from God. Unfortunately, that's not the case. Nevertheless, I've come a long way toward healing. I don't sit and constantly cry to my Father in pain, wishing for the end of my existence. I don't need my children to dig their fingernails into my feet every day to get some feeling back in them. I don't need someone to sit on my chest anymore to try to relieve the discomfort. I don't need to take off my glasses continuously throughout the day to give my eyes some relief, and I rarely have eye problems where I lose my sight.

I no longer get pneumonia every winter, and I no longer need to (or even desire to) lie down all the time because I'm in so much pain. My leg no longer drags when I walk, and my hair no longer falls out of my head and my lower legs. I'm calling this list of things no longer happening "improvements," and there are even more than the ones I've listed here. Above everything else, I prayed for God to keep me alive long enough to see my kids grow into adults, and I am blessed and grateful that He allowed me to do just that.

Complete healing, however, hasn't yet occurred. To be honest, it can get discouraging at times to realize this—especially because I'd felt, at least at one point in time, that if I'd follow God's command to put everything down on paper, He would wrap things up with a bang by giving me back my health. Apparently, He has other plans.

I wish I could say I've responded in a godly way, peacefully submitting to His will without doubts or contention, but I haven't. Instead, I've been grieving. My heart has cried out more than once in despair. *Haven't I had enough faith in You, Lord? Haven't I shown You enough love? Why won't You heal me?*

Although I've not been healed, I recognize how my environment and my choices—or those made by others for me and not by God—have been responsible for some of my health issues. Way back as an infant, for example, my mom's decision to use formula rather than breastmilk for my nourishment placed my body at a disadvantage.

Another incident that negatively affected my health as a child was my exposure to antibiotics during a hospital stay at age four. Sure, my life was in danger at that point, and this may have ultimately saved my life. I've been told, however, that it's likely to have negatively impacted my stomach flora and created a leaky gut that some believe may be responsible for so many of my other health challenges, and especially because I took a heavy dose of antibiotics again in my late forties in an attempt to manage the chronic Lyme disease.

Still, another choice with negative results was my decision to work at a plastics thermoforming plant for over twenty-nine years (a place where, thankfully, I no longer work). Someone once suggested that the surface of my intestines resembled a rubber tube, which logically seems related to many years of working with PVC and HIPS plastics during my time there. If true, this would obviously make it difficult for nutrients to pass from food into my system and, thus, for my body to utilize what I eat to keep me healthy.

Some things, though, haven't been choices, especially during my childhood years. One is a negative self-image. For as long as I can remember, I've been contending with a disagreeable inner voice that has affected the way I look at myself, those around me, and my world as a whole. Even now, as an adult, although I am more capable of challenging that negativity, it's been a constant struggle. In both cases, it's safe to say that such negativity has affected my mental health and ultimately caused issues with my physical health, as well.

Another issue that has affected me is my temperament. I've been a highly emotional person all my life. As a result, my body has been producing and cycling incredibly high levels of cortisol through my system since I was very, very young. The cortisol has depleted my adrenals and wreaked havoc with my organs, further weakening my already-challenged body.

Overall, I've experienced a lot of misfortune in my life, and for many years, I was more than a little irritated at God for this. Why was He ignoring my pleas for better health? Over the years, however, as my faith has deepened and my awareness of my situation has been clarified, I've realized that none of the things that have made me sick were God's fault. All of these things—lack of nutrients from breastfeeding, overuse of antibiotics, ingestion of plastics residues, toxic negativity, and a highly sensitive temperament—all of these things were caused by man. While God allowed them, He did not cause them. It makes me wonder if what Jesus said about the blind man in John 9:3 might have related to me, too: "Jesus answered, 'It was neither that this man sinned, nor his parents; but it was so that the works of God might be displayed in him.'"

The health challenges I have faced throughout my life have helped me connect with that blind man. Regardless of what has caused my struggles, I recognize that I, too, can be a vessel for displaying the works of God. How I cope now and in the future can shine a light on my love for Him and His love for me. I want to be that man.

With this in mind, I've tried for quite some time to hide my disappointment with the struggles I've faced and acted as though I was stronger than the pain, even when it was almost overwhelming. With God's grace, I've done a pretty good job most of the time. Even so, I allowed myself to be beaten on too many occasions. I complained, was grumpy, or used critical words toward those around me who I felt weren't doing enough to help me.

One night, after an especially difficult time when I felt Mary wasn't giving me nearly enough respect for all I struggled with each day, she blurted something out in frustration that was especially hurtful to me. It was also, though, quite possibly, just what I needed. It was something she'd been considering for quite a while but didn't know how to say, and she didn't want to hurt my feelings and cause a divide between us that might be too deep to bridge. Mary told me that one of the specialists I'd seen had told her that working with me was a difficult task because, she felt, I was consumed by a "victim mentality." In fact, when Mary requested another appointment for me with her, she was told that it wouldn't be beneficial because I simply did not want to get better; that I'd rather be a victim than be in good health and assume the responsibility that came with good health.

When Mary heard this, she asked another of my healers about the situation. Although that woman used a slightly gentler tone, she agreed and explained that my body wasn't healing largely because of the state of my mind. Mary then recalled the words of a counselor we'd visited several years ago who, when Mary asked her if my pattern of thinking was irrational, replied affirmatively, stating that this was true "without a doubt."

I don't know if I was more upset by Mary's apparent belief in this concept or by the idea that so many others felt this way about me. I thought, *how dare they be so thoughtless!* I caught myself, however, and somehow accepted that these words could be true—at least somewhat and on some occasions.

Despite the fact that Mary's words and the opinions of the others pierced me deeply, God must have given me enough grace in the moment to consider them because I worked them through my mind for many weeks. One of the first things I did was clarify the message. The specialists weren't hinting that I had chosen to become infected with the Lyme disease bacteria or that at age four, I'd be admitted to the hospital where life-saving antibiotics had been administered. Nor were they hinting that shortly afterward, I'd chosen to develop an extreme reaction to hay fever and later to so many other things.

What these people were expressing, however, was that because I'd lived with anxiety, depression, and personal insecurity for so long—unconsciously for most of the time, but with more awareness in later years—I'd compromised my immune system and my own personal resolve for physical, emotional, and mental well-being. They were saying that while I might not have been responsible for the initial cause of my health problems, my continued negative thinking was toxic and that it was standing in the way of good health.

Some might wonder how a person with as much love for God

as I had would have such a poor outlook on life. It wasn't that I didn't love God with all my heart. I did—more and more each year. The problem, as I see it now, is that I'd always felt that God didn't love me. Certainly, He loved me enough to create me, to create a world for me to live in, and to feed and clothe me. Even so, it didn't feel like He really loved me as unique, as someone special. After all, He had planned for me to be the eighth child, born to older parents who were too tired to provide the emotional care I needed. He had allowed me to struggle in school so much that many of my classmates picked on me, and my teachers gave up on me. He permitted my older brother to dominate and continually bully me. Moreover, for all of these years, He has allowed me, despite day after day after day of pleading for healing, to remain sick—and increasingly so—almost throughout my entire life. I guess you could say that I was a half-Christian—I was allowing the love intended to fill my life to flow in only one direction. I recognize now that this is simply not enough!

God's love must be allowed to go both ways!

To help me better understand and become immersed in the idea of God's love for me, Mary suggested I start listening to affirmations. Affirmations are repeated words or sentences that express a positive message meant to flood your subconscious with healthy thoughts. They are like the best parents coaching you every morning or evening about how you should think and about how to manage your way through life's complications. When I started listening to affirmations, I almost instantly recognized that this new voice in my head was vastly different from the one I'd had there for much of my life. Over time, I'd let the struggles I'd faced turn my mind into a dry, brittle landscape that was barren of hope and joy. The affirmations were like a gentle rain that refreshed that soil, bringing back contentment, peace, and faith.

The first affirmations I listened to focused on the topic of joy. I found the topic after a short YouTube search, then put on my earphones and played it on loop while I slept. When I awoke the next day, I was pleasantly surprised at how peaceful I felt—a condition that lasted much of the day. Buoyed by these positive vibes, I began to consider how affirmations could be used to help my attitude in other ways. My mind eventually wandered to the concept of physical health. Might affirmations be available to help me condition my brain into believing it was healed, change my attitude, or even somehow, actually heal my body of the issues I had been struggling with for so long? After all, Romans 10:17 says, "So faith comes from hearing, and hearing by the word of Christ."

That evening, I looked up "healing affirmations" and discovered more than I could ever have imagined. I couldn't wait to give them a try.

Some of the affirmations I found were short, but others were nearly an hour long. I selected one of the longer ones, put in my earphones, and began to listen. I was thrilled to discover that most of the healing videos weren't just positive words about my health but that they also incorporated words from The Divine—Biblical passages of hope and healing. I immediately felt an overwhelming sense of God's presence, which makes sense in light of Philippians 4:8-9:

> Finally, brothers *and sisters*, whatever is true, whatever is honorable, whatever is right, whatever is pure, whatever is lovely, whatever is commendable, if there is any excellence and if anything worthy of praise, think about these things. As for the things you have learned and received and heard and seen in me, practice these things, and the God of peace will be with you.

In addition to the comfort I felt from the Biblical references in the affirmations I'd chosen, I was reminded of how often Jesus spoke about healing, and when I read or listened to those parts of the Bible, I was struck by how many times faith was connected to healing. Consider the following examples:

> When the woman whose daughter was tormented by demons cried out to Jesus for mercy, He responded: "O woman, your faith is great; it shall be done for you as you desire." And her daughter was healed at once.
> Matthew 15:28

> When the Roman centurion asked Jesus to speak a word of healing for his paralyzed servant, Jesus responded: "Truly I say to you, I have not found such great faith with anyone in Israel. And I say to you that many will come from east and west, and recline *at the table* with Abraham, Isaac, and Jacob in the kingdom of heaven; but the sons of the kingdom will be thrown out into the outer darkness; in that place there will be weeping and gnashing of teeth." And

> Jesus said to the centurion, "Go; it shall be done for you as you have believed." And the servant was healed at that *very* moment.
> Mathew 8:10-13

> To the woman who had been long-inflicted with bleeding, who wanted to simply touch the edge of Jesus' cloak, He replied: "Daughter, take courage; your faith has made you well." And at once the woman was made well.
> Matthew 9:22

> When a man's friends lowered him through the roof into the home where Jesus taught, seeing their faith, He said: "Friend, your sins are forgiven you."
> Luke 5:20

> When two blind men called out to Jesus to take pity on them, who replied that they had faith that Jesus could heal them, He touched their eyes, saying: "It shall be done for you according to your faith."
> Matthew 9:29

Many times in the Bible, Jesus healed the sick without requiring anything from them. In other verses, though, the people were told to take some kind of action to bring about healing. This was true with Mary and Martha when they asked for Jesus' help after their brother Lazarus had died:

> So Jesus, again being deeply moved within, came to the tomb. Now it was a cave, and a stone was lying against it. Jesus said, "Remove the stone." Martha, the sister of the deceased, said to Him, "Lord, by this time there will be a stench, for he has been *dead* four days." Jesus said to her, "Did I not say to you that if you believe, you will see the glory of God?" So they removed the stone. And Jesus raised His eyes, and said, "Father, I thank You that You have heard Me. But I knew that You always hear Me; nevertheless, because of the people standing around I said *it*, so that they may believe that You sent Me." And when He had said these things, He cried out with a loud voice, "Lazarus, come out!" Out came the man who had died, bound hand and foot with wrappings, and his face was wrapped around with a cloth. Jesus said to them, "Unbind him, and let him go."
> John 11:38-44

I began to wonder what additional things God might be asking of me to instigate healing. I knew, of course, that faith itself was the key. Perhaps, though, I needed to do other things for it to occur, even if it meant simply talking to and then listening for His response about what might be needed for me to heal.

These two factors, then, took center stage in my mind: healing brought about through faith and conversation with Him about what else He wished me to do. So I started to plan how I might be called to use faith and action in my own healing journey. Like me, the people in the Bible who had been cured by Jesus had often suffered for many years before they were healed. Perhaps they had been showing a little faith for most of that time, or perhaps it grew over time or even just swelled up in them one day when they saw Jesus. Regardless, one day they were healed, and it appeared this had occurred only because of their faith. I know now I must have that faith too, and I must both believe it in my heart and show it with my words and actions.

In addition to having and showing faith, I also must not just sit around and wait for healing. I have to actively seek it. I can't just fall on my knees each night and plead for help. I can't just lie around on the couch thinking about what might be wrong and how it got that way. I have to get up, think positively, and take good care of my body and my mind. When one thing doesn't work, I have to proceed ahead to find another. I have to participate in my healing—not just wait around for it. This is shown in James 2:14-17:

> What use is it, my brothers *and sisters*, if someone says he has faith, but he has no works? Can that faith save him? If a brother or sister is without clothing and in need of daily food, and one of you says to them, "Go in peace, be warmed and be filled," yet you do not give them what is necessary for *their* body, what use is that? In the same way, faith also, if it has no works, is dead, *being* by itself.

Before I started listening to affirmations, the amount of time I spent thinking about my problems only served to strengthen them because my thoughts were always so negative. I continually evaluated how I was feeling, how today's feelings compared to yesterday's, and what this might mean for me later today, tomorrow, next week, or next year. What had gone wrong in my childhood to set me off on this wrong path, what systems were not working in my body, why did most doctors seem to have so little consideration for my condition, etc.? Between feeling anger at my situation and trying to work out a solution, obsessing over my health almost never stopped.

Now I know that if I'm serious about improving my health, I

have to go all in to eliminate any negative thinking that could be getting in the way. So I am making a conscious effort to give less attention to my illness, which is definitely easier said than done. For example, when I'm at home with time to think, I try not to lie around pondering my challenges but instead get up and focus on the positive words I've heard when listening to affirmations.

Some of the effects of my new mindset have paid off very quickly. For example, I am much more calm and positive after listening to affirmations. Alternatively, I can be short-tempered and easily overwhelmed when I go a few days without listening to them. I am starting to see my challenges as just a part of me—not the whole of me. Some days it is easier than others, but I know that this has to be my mindset for me to feel better and to be healed.

These days, I typically fill my head with positive things whenever I get the chance. I listen to healing Bible verses, sermons, hymns, healing frequencies, and affirmations. I watch wholesome TV shows like *The Waltons* and *Leave It to Beaver*. I envision a God who loves me as a unique and special being. I try not to speak or even think about dietary sacrifice or physical difficulties. I work really hard to dismiss disappointments instead of brooding over them. I release thoughts that previously would have entangled me in hours of reasoning without resolution. I also strive to ignore the inner voice that tells me I am not feeling well enough to do something or that I don't have the energy I need to get something done. My conscious self knows God wants all of us to be healthy, happy, confident, and successful, and I am working hard to engrain this understanding into my subconscious. I no longer want just to pray and hope for the best. I want—and now work—to really trust Him.

I am moving forward in a very positive and godly way. I truly love Him with all my heart, mind, soul, and might. I always have. As painful and miserable as I've often let my life become, I wouldn't dream of changing the closeness I've developed with Him as a result of my struggles. Sometimes I've had a good attitude about life, and other times a less than positive one, but my love for God has never wavered—and it never will. I may not know God's specific intentions for my future, but I am confident they are pure and good. I know God loves me, and I will cling to

Him no matter what challenges lie ahead. I pray that my story will convince others to do the same.

I pray that whatever struggle or suffering you may be facing, the Lord reveals His love to you and His desire for your healing. Meditate on His Word, and I promise you will feel better. Who knows, you may even be completely healed.

God bless,

John

Printed in the USA
CPSIA information can be obtained
at www.ICGtesting.com
LVHW081505211223
766988LV00096B/5413